TROUBLE SPOT FAT LOSS

D1280143

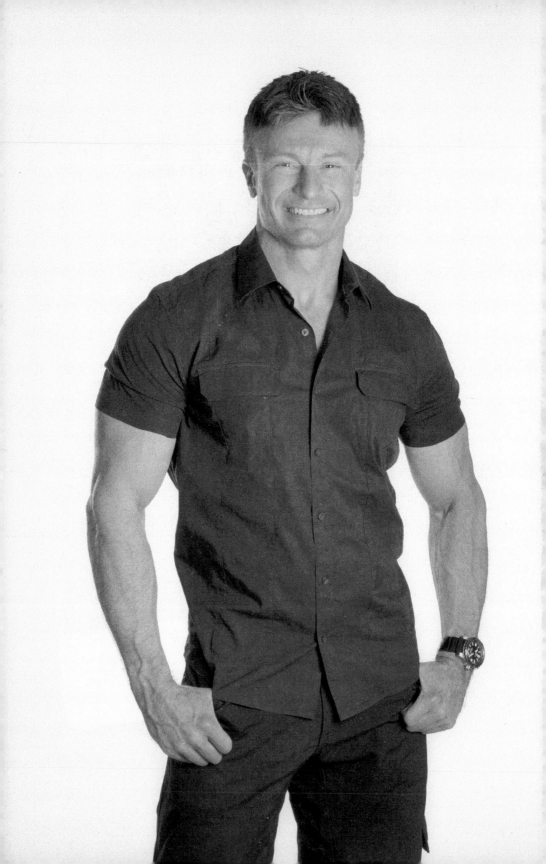

TROUBLE SPOT FAT LOSS

LOSE WEIGHT, BUILD MUSCLE, & SAY GOODBYE to PROBLEM AREAS FOR GOOD

BRUCE KRAHN

appetite

by RANDOM HOUSE

Copyright © 2015 Bruce Krahn

All rights reserved. The use of any part of this publication, reproduced, transmitted in any form or by any means electronic, mechanical, photocopying, recording or otherwise, or stored in a retrieval system without the prior written consent of the publisher—or in the case of photocopying or other reprographic copying, license from the Canadian Copyright Licensing Agency—is an infringement of the copyright law.

Appetite by Random House® is a registered trademark of Random House LLC.

Library and Archives of Canada Cataloguing in Publication
is available upon request.

Print ISBN: 978-0-449-01653-4
eBook ISBN: 978-0-449-01654-1

Cover image: Grant Hickey, except front cover top middle © Lior Zilberstein / Stocksy United, top right © Lumina / Stocksy United
Cover and book design by Five Seventeen
Printed and bound in the USA

Image on page 180 appears courtesy of *Revive* magazine.

Published in Canada by Appetite by Random House®,
A division of Random House of Canada Limited,
A Penguin Random House Company

www.penguinrandomhouse.ca

10 9 8 7 6 5 4 3 2 1

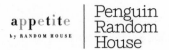

CONTENTS

Part Three—Your Body Minus the Fat

Part Four—Your Body Plus the Muscle

Recipes

Exercises

TROUBLE
SPOT
FAT
LOSS

FOREWORD

The book you are holding in your hands contains the most cutting-edge, valid, and effective advice for losing trouble spot fat than anything else on the market today. If you've tried to lose fat and failed, you've probably figured out that more than 90% of diet and fitness advice out there is not just bad, it's dead wrong.

"Eat less, move more" has been the most overhyped mantra of the past 50 years. I've found it interesting that despite this idea being pushed by a lot of fitness and diet "gurus" and even by medical doctors, in those 50 years we've witnessed the biggest spike in obesity in history.

"Eat less, move more" is simply bad advice. Next time you hear it, turn around and run. It's the advice of simpletons, armchair experts, and the uneducated. Most offer this advice in a breezy spirit of brushing off complications and trying to "keep things simple."

Staying in shape is not that simple. If it were, such a high percentage of the population wouldn't be obese. However, rest assured it's not overly complicated either. But it does require science, a sound strategy, and sustainability, as you'll soon see.

The problem with the "eat less" part of the mantra is that eating less will make you hungry, kill your energy to burn fat, and strip away any and all of your calorie-burning, optimal body-shaping lean muscle. It will simply back your body into a corner, with nowhere to go.

Let's say I eat 2000 calories a day, and I'm overweight. So I "eat less" by cutting down to 1500 calories a day. I lose weight briefly before my metabolism adjusts by slowing down, and I regain most of the weight back.

So, what do I do when my old "less" becomes the new "more" and I start to gain weight again? Go down to 1000 calories? When does that stop? There is no limit to the notion of "eat less," which officially makes this the worst advice. Ever.

Similarly, the problem with the "move more" part of the mantra is that there is no measurability or end point. Do I keep going until I hurt myself? Until I win an Olympic gold medal? Until I'm living at the gym, working out two hours a day?

The mantra simply suggests move more, but it provides no stopping point. There's no "until." When pressed, "experts" who espouse this mantra will say that "move more" entails going to the gym on a regular basis and being active throughout the day. It might mean taking the stairs instead of the elevator, choosing a parking spot that's further from the door, and so on.

And aren't you already doing this? And where has it got you? The problem is that this advice does not include intensity, effort, or progression—the cornerstone components of great health and a body others envy.

Sure, the "move more" advice may help you lose the first 10 or 20 pounds of body fat if you're lucky, but it'll never help you lose those final pounds of trouble spot fat hiding your sexy and sculpted frame underneath.

I assume the unspoken finish line for the "Eat less, move more" mantra is reaching your target weight. But what if you never reach it? Or what if you hit it but look soft, scrawny, and weak? Or what if you hit it by following unsustainable diet and fitness habits that ruin your social life? Well, I guess it's just a matter of time before you gain all that weight back and blame yourself for not being able to follow this "simple" advice.

So, what's the solution?

Before I get into that, let me share my personal experience. As a bestselling muscle-building author and professional fitness model, I believe in effective training. I was strongly nudged by a close friend, the famous Dr. John Berardi, to link up with Bruce because he was on to some cutting-edge information to eliminate trouble spot fat, and it was very different from what the mainstream media and magazines were teaching. I had to know more, since I always have a hard time losing the final few pounds around my lower abs. And I wanted to use the information to look and feel my best and pass it on to my clients who struggled with trouble spots of their own, such as the lower back, chest, thighs, triceps, and butt.

Bruce and I met at my favorite Mediterranean restaurant, and it was immediately apparent that he was the real deal. I couldn't help but size him up in between bites of my chicken and tabbouleh. Forty-five years old, he was ripped to shreds with bulging biceps and a physique that dripped with confidence, and if not for his genuine and grateful smile, I would have been intimidated.

The purpose of our meet-up was to discuss his desire to grow his online business—my expertise. He told me about his debilitating bout of depression that almost ended his life in his early 20s. How he turned to dumbbells and barbells instead of drugs, and how these events led to a turning point in his life that resulted in a career in fitness. Helping others with fitness and diet just clicked for him, and shortly after he found himself busy in the world of celebrity training with the likes of Nelly Furtado, Criss Angel, and Tom Cochrane.

Did I say I was impressed?

I was most impressed that Bruce's physique represented a "trade up"—and that means a lot coming from a guy who is a world-class fitness model and hangs out with many of the greatest fitness models and bodybuilders in the world.

Truth is, in my world, the majority of fitness and diet "gurus" are a joke. We laugh at them because they preach one thing and do another, and most of them fall into two physique categories: skinny and weak, or soft and chubby. Personally, I don't take advice from people who don't look the part—I don't care how many academic degrees they have listed after their name. Don't export your advice if it's not working in your own life!

Like I said, Bruce is the real deal. He practices what he preaches and wears the medal of all medals: six-pack abs 365 days a year, not just when it's time to get ready for a photo shoot. I understand that not everyone wants six-pack abs, but if you're going to give fat-loss advice, at least have a flat stomach!

I asked him, "Bruce, what's your approach to getting rid of trouble spot body fat—you know, those last 10 to 20 pounds of stubborn fat?" And that's when he told me about his brand-new masterpiece, *Trouble Spot Fat Loss*.

As someone who gets pitched dozens of "new" product ideas, rarely does anything truly new come across my desk. I asked him, "What makes *Trouble Spot Fat Loss* different from the other gazillion diet books out there?"

Bruce replied, "This is the only book that specifically addresses the problem of losing gender-specific trouble spot fat. While there are plenty of books on weight loss, there is no book that specifically speaks to the hormonal cause of hard-to-lose fat in problem areas, and what can be done to get rid of it."

I let out a huge sigh of relief. I might have thrown the rest of my chicken at him if he had said "It's simple, just move more and eat less . . ."

Trouble Spot Fat Loss is a scientific approach to reducing fat around your personal trouble spots, using innovative and amazingly effective methods to help both the athletic and the not-so-athletic.

Bruce explained that the reason so many people have trouble spots is imbalances in their body's biochemistry, especially imbalances of hormones. If you doubt the power of hormones, take a look at what steroids have done to so many athletes. And just as steroid hormones can build muscle, other hormones can cause you to store fat on your belly, back, legs, hips, and arms. His approach is beyond super-cool and explains why the entire "Eat less, move more" mantra fails so many hardworking, good folks.

Not only does *Trouble Spot Fat Loss* educate you on what really matters when it comes to overall fat loss but it gives fitness-focused individuals an edge—something to take their results to the next level. If you already train hard, belong to a fitness club, purchase organic food, regularly consume supplements, and are out for getting great results, this is *the* book missing from your fitness library.

Bruce teaches you scientific, strategic, and sustainable methods to take your body to its optimal physique, without all the unwanted fat. Apply his carb-fasting regimen (see chapter 7) and Adrenaline Protocols (see chapter 8) and you'll shock your friends the next time you strip down to your bathing suit at a pool party. They'll all want to know what you've been up to.

Bruce shows you how to shed your trouble fat, and keep it off. Then it's all about your body plus the muscle. This is where every other book fails, and becomes just the next diet book.

Unless you learn how to add at least 10 pounds of muscle to your body, you will forever struggle to lose fat. End of story. Adding a few pounds of lean calorie-burning muscle is the ultimate answer to permanent fat loss and to balancing and optimizing your hormones.

Without this information, kiss your dreams of ever having a sexy, attention-grabbing body that commands respect goodbye. You will lose the fat and put it back on, and then repeat the cycle, for the rest of your life. Despite your efforts, you'll live the rest of your life looking average at best. Follow Bruce's carb-feasting advice for the fastest way to gain 10 pounds of muscle, and your life will never be the same again.

With the common bond of achieving optimal health, fitness, and performance, Bruce and I intuitively understood one another. As an Internet marketing pro, I immediately knew I wanted to help Bruce spread his message throughout the world, and I wanted to support him with the most ethical and compelling marketing strategies to beat up the "bad guys" who serve up garbage advice.

Our professional relationship grew out of that lunch meeting, and the rest is history.

Trouble Spot Fat Loss is a gold mine of cutting-edge information that will help you to understand why we store body fat in certain areas. Bruce's is a step-by-step system. There isn't a smarter, easier, or more comprehensive system out there. If you're looking for a real approach to eliminate trouble spot fat and to keep it off, this is it. I'm also confident that, in addition to the extraordinary results, you'll enjoy the process immensely—just as I have, and the clients I've passed this information along to.

Be bold, live large, make things happen.

Vince Del Monte
Hamilton, Canada

Why the heck would I want to write a fitness book?

This is the question I was asked at least a dozen times before I began assembling the information—a conglomeration of thoughts, theories, experiments, and research—that you now hold in your hands.

After all, writing a book is no simple task. Often it takes at least two years of dedicated work from start to finish, all in the hope that once it is published, people will actually read it. But, for me, there was a bigger reason—the information I wanted to share wasn't just about how the strategies I had developed could help people look fantastic and perform at their best; this was also, when it really came down to it, the story about how exercise and nutrition actually saved my life . . . twice.

I grew up the middle of three boys in a working-class family. I had your typical Canadian Prairie childhood, including dreams of playing in the NHL and living someplace warm in the winter. What wasn't typical was my perspective on life and how I fit into this world. Starting at around the age of 12, I began to struggle with low self-esteem and depression. I really should have become an actor, since for most of my young life I was able to hide these feelings from the people around me, never seeking help. I rationalized that everybody felt the same way and that I should therefore simply bury my feelings and get on with my life.

As any therapist will tell you, suppressing your feelings will only buy time for so long, and at one point or another you will have to face your demons. For me, the showdown with my demons came in the spring of 1988 when I was hit with a bout of depression that led me to the brink of taking my own life.

Having suffered from clinical depression, I can tell you one thing for certain: there is little anybody can say that will suddenly make a clinically depressed person feel better. I actually avoided situations where I might be subjected to some form of amateur (or even professional) psychoanalysis. I felt like crap, didn't see any point to life, and wasn't interested in hearing about how great my life really was or how much people loved me. For me, being depressed was a solitary existence—like being a lone man clinging to a life preserver in the middle of an ocean of despair . . . and I was getting tired of hanging on. I was 19 years old and I was done with the whole living thing.

MY BREAKTHROUGH

To appease my mother, I finally sought the council of a psychiatrist who specialized in depression and suicidal teenagers. His treatment plan was simple: take Prozac and meet with him once or twice a month to talk about my feelings. Just what every young man wants—drugs that make you sleepy and kill your sex drive, and long drawn-out discussions about your feelings. But I was game if he was and so began my experience with psychotropic drugs and talk therapy.

This lasted all of two weeks. I hated being on Prozac—it made me sleepy all the time and feel totally confused. And talking about my deepest feelings just made me feel worse about who I was. This treatment plan was clearly not going to work, and I began to retreat into the dark thoughts that had become my default.

It was at this time that I decided to revisit exercising. I remember looking in the mirror and being really upset by what I saw. The past year of inactivity, poor appetite, and self-destructive behavior had left my body looking more like that of an old Arnold Palmer than a young Arnold Schwarzenegger. I had played around with training before but never took it seriously. But I had enjoyed being in the gym and exercising with weights. We have all heard stories of people having epiphanies, moments of extreme clarity that serve as personal revelations and breakthroughs, and that is exactly what I had.

I can vividly recall sitting in my car in the gym's parking lot with my head full of my usual dark thoughts. It was then that I had my epiphany and made a promise to myself—I would substitute pumping iron for Prozac. I was acutely aware how exercise improved my mental as well as physical functioning, and I knew that with each workout I would feel at least 1% better. And so for the next 12 months I lived for that 1%. Against the advice of my doctor, I took myself off Prozac and immersed myself in getting better.

I ate healthier food.
I trained consistently.
I got more sleep.
I read more books.

It may sound clichéd, but this one decision changed the entire course of my life. Exercise and nutrition gave me what the drugs and psychoanalysis couldn't—my life back. This decision heavily influenced all future decisions I made, including to pursue fitness as a career, and to write and share my story. Looking back, I can say that this experience made me a much better coach, as I have firsthand understanding of one of the toughest and least talked about aspects of the human experience: mental illness.

And that wasn't to be the only time exercise and nutrition saved my life. The second time came some 20 years later when I found my health failing fast in the midst of a personal and professional meltdown that left me broken once again. The difference was that this time I was older and the symptoms were physical, not psychological. You will read about what happened in chapter 10, but suffice to say that I found myself in desperate need of physical transformation. The techniques I used to rehabilitate myself are discussed in detail in that chapter.

Life is the greatest teacher of all, and these trials have made me who I am today—a husband, father, friend, trainer, and teacher with a tremendous wealth of knowledge about how the human body functions, what it can endure, and how it can be transformed mentally and physically. I encourage you to keep the knowledge that you and your body have the capacity to change in mind as you read the following pages and embark on your own journey of transformation.

INTRODUCTION

Rachel was *not* happy. In fact, she was downright pissed off.

"What the hell is going on here, Bruce? I am exercising five times per week and eating nothing but carrots and cauliflower, and still I have these annoying saddlebags!"

Her husband let out a snicker and lifted his shirt to admire his newfound best friend—his now-visible abs. "Maybe it was that biscotti you had last week. At the rate I'm going, I'll be going shirtless to work on a regular basis."

But Rachel wasn't laughing, and for good reason. After all, she had given up so much lately in her endeavor to lose those saddlebags:

No alcohol
No bread
No chocolate
No *fun*

On top of this, she was working out like (as she described it) a "fat-obsessed, crazed lunatic."

It's not as though I hadn't seen this before. Quite the contrary, in fact. Over the past two decades, I have witnessed this type of frustration more times than I can count, and I am firmly convinced that *women and men are* not *created equal*.

Now, hold on a second—before you dismiss me as being some sort of throwback, allow me to explain.

There truly are many differences between the sexes. We dress differently. We sound different. Generally, we look different and like different things. From the time we are born we are taught to behave differently. Advertising agencies are aware of this and market their clients' products and services differently depending on which sex they are trying to appeal to.

In terms of physiology, men and women are different as well. Our internal and external biological systems are not the same. These systems determine how our bodies respond to various forms of stimuli, including what we eat and how we exercise. Nowhere is the difference between the sexes more obvious than in the realm of body fat distribution: men and women store and metabolize fat differently from each other.

Most women are likely to be carrying more fat than the average man. And not only do they have more of it but they are also far more efficient at storing it. When a woman gains fat, she will usually store it in the lower body, particularly in the hips, butt, and legs. This differs from the average man, who is more likely to gain fat in the upper body, usually around the belly, chest, and love handles. As well as storing fat in different places, men and women store different types of fat. Men are more likely to build up visceral fat—the deadly type that surrounds internal organs—while women are more likely to develop subcutaneous fat, which is a form of white fat that feels squishy and is located just underneath the skin.

In terms of health, women who carry more fat than average are better off than men who do the same. The typical lower-body fat distribution found on a woman may actually be indicative of robust hormonal health, whereas abdominal fat on a man suggests quite the opposite. A man with the stereotypical beer belly may be at risk for various health conditions, including insulin resistance and diabetes.

Women and men also burn fat differently. When a woman burns fat, she loses it from her upper body first, and from the lower body last. In some cases, a woman will lose fat from her upper body and even achieve visible abdominal muscles while her lower body remains unchanged. The exact opposite is true for most men, who will often have ripped thighs and calves while still sporting an impressive beer belly. This is the fat I am referring to when I talk about trouble spot fat—those pounds and inches that are the hardest to lose.

There is one primary evolutionary reason for these differences between men and women: reproduction. A woman's body is designed to carry and foster the healthy development of future offspring. Her body is programmed to store in the form of fat the energy and nutrients needed to support another life for months at a time. These powerful biological signals have no interest in or concern with a woman's desire to look a particular way and will gladly override any attempts to get rid of this stored fat, even if she is in a calorie deficit.

Men, therefore, have it much easier when it comes to losing trouble spot fat. A man's biological contribution to future offspring is brief and minimal at best—all he has to do is fertilize a woman's egg. His body is programmed to lose fat more easily. A woman's body has a whole lot more to be concerned with.

THIS BOOK IS *NOT* ABOUT SPOT REDUCTION

The term "spot reduction" refers to the idea that you can burn fat preferentially in one area over another. This is a notion perpetuated by late-night infomercials trying to sell you various abdominal-targeted exercise gadgets that supposedly significantly reduce fat from that area alone.

From a big-picture standpoint, spot reduction is a myth. A man with 40% body fat and a 42-inch waist cannot simply perform 100 crunches per day and expect to lose fat from only his midsection. Nor can a woman tell her body to lose fat only from her thighs while sparing the fat in her chest. (Sorry!)

Fat loss is by and large systemic, and your body will reduce body fat stores from the easiest places to do so first, and from the more difficult trouble spots last. If a person begins a weight-loss program and loses fat from only one area of the body, it is simply because this is what their body was preprogrammed to do. However, as you are about to discover, *you can influence the efficiency with which fat is lost from, and muscle is gained in, your trouble spots.*

Since your body will shed easy-to-lose fat first, pretty much any non-ridiculous diet will work in the beginning. The methods described in this book will help you reduce your body fat and ultimately get to the level where you can address your trouble spots. If you have yet to shed the "easy-to-lose" fat, start out by following the recommendations outlined in chapter 1, then get ready to implement the more advanced methods described in this book. Although no one can change genetically predetermined patterns of body fat loss, these methods will facilitate the shedding of your most diet-and-exercise-resistant body fat stores without sacrificing muscle tissue along the way.

IT'S NOT *JUST* ABOUT LOSING FAT

I have spent the better part of the past two decades researching and then applying various diet, training, and supplements regimens to a diverse range of clients, as well as to myself. I have experimented with different food combinations, meal timing, calorie cycling, carb cycling, carb loading, carb restriction, fasting, protein cycling, and megadoses of supplements and vitamins—and even various prescription medications. I have treated (and mistreated) my body to exercise regimens ranging from one hour a week to three hours a day, and experimented with every advanced training technique known to man. All this I did with one quest in mind: finding the most efficient way to achieve optimal body composition in the fastest possible time. In other words, I've been asking, what is the best method for losing fat while maintaining (or even increasing) lean body mass?

And I have found the answer. You are about to discover how to achieve ridiculous, jaw-dropping results in record time with the least amount of effort. As you apply these techniques, you will also become a better athlete and a person who no longer makes excuses—you'll be a person who makes things happen instead.

PART ONE
FUNDAMENTALS

1

Small Hinges Swing Big Doors

14 Essential Rules for Body Transformation

Humans are driven by curiosity, and it is simply human nature to want to know a secret. In my practice, I have often been pressed by clients to let them in on what my secret is to staying lean and muscular year-round. When I tell them what the "secret" is, they are usually disappointed. I think they would rather hear that I take some exotic herb, or one I found growing under my back porch or something. But it's nothing like that. Rather, it's a step-by-step approach. And whether it be in business, relationships, or body transformation, it is always best to start with actionable steps that produce the biggest result for the least amount of expenditure of time, money, and effort. Anything else will simply overcomplicate things and leave you feeling confused and frustrated, and ultimately cause you to quit.

Author, philanthropist, and businessman W. Clement Stone once said, "Small hinges swing big doors." Given his wise words, I can only assume that Mr. Stone had fantastic abs. There are 14 such "hinges" that serve to increase our muscle mass, decrease body fat, and improve physical performance. If you are just beginning your body recomposition journey, I insist that you follow the 14 essential rules outlined below, as they lay the foundation for some of my voodoo-magic body-transformation techniques described in the coming chapters.

RULE 1: EAT FEWER CALORIES THAN YOU BURN

Creating a calorie deficit is the single most important factor to losing body fat. There are three ways in which this can be done: eat fewer calories, increase calorie expenditure through exercise, or do a combination of the two. Because of the body's response to exercise, which you will learn about in the coming pages, I always recommend the latter of the three. But don't make the mistake of assuming that you will have to carry around a little scale to measure your food with. Such OCD behavior is neither necessary nor realistic. Instead, for the time being, simply focus on eating less food Monday through Friday and letting loose a bit on the weekends. This will prepare you nicely for implementing what you will learn when we discuss food choices and planning meals.

For those who wish to run the numbers, use this formula to calculate your daily calorie intake:

Your body weight in pounds × 10 kcal = daily calorie intake

Your calorie intake will likely fluctuate, unless you eat the same exact things every day. Just try to keep the number to within 10% of the calculation, whether over or under. You'll learn more about calorie counting and the chart that follows in chapter 7.

In the meantime, here are a few calculations for fat-loss calorie intake, along with the 10% variable range.

Fat-Loss Calorie Guide

BODY WEIGHT	DAILY CALORIE INTAKE (-/+ 10% RANGE)
100 lb	1000 kcal (900–1100)
150 lb	1500 kcal (1350–1650)
200 lb	2000 kcal (1800–2200)
250 lb	2500 kcal (2250–2750)
300 lb	3000 kcal (2700–3300)

RULE 2: EAT FEWER PROCESSED FOODS

Chronic overconsumption of high-calorie foods with low nutrient content is a recipe for increased hunger, food cravings, and increased body fat. While it is important that your diet predominantly consists of nutrient-rich foods, this does not mean you can *never* eat processed food. Thinking that you will never again enjoy pizza, french fries, or the occasional donut is unrealistic and completely unnecessary. In the following chapters you'll learn how you can incorporate *any* food into your diet each week and still lose fat from your trouble spots.

The issue I have with processed and refined foods is that most lack in nutrient value and yet are high in calories and trans fats. They are filled with additives, taste enhancers, sugar, artificial sweeteners, preservatives, and loads of chemicals we can hardly pronounce let alone digest. All these additives disrupt our hormonal balance, and leave our cells deprived of nutrients. Even some foods traditionally thought to be healthy, such as rice, pasta, and bread, are typically overprocessed. These foods have often been refined or stripped of their fiber and nutrient content, bleached, and packaged for a long shelf life. Overconsumption can lead to many health problems, including weight gain, digestive problems, fatigue, hypoglycemia, and skin disorders.

FOODS TO ELIMINATE

- All white baked goods—muffins (even bran muffins, folks!), cakes, cookies, white bread, donuts
- Processed cereals, granola bars
- Refined grains—white pasta, quick-cooking oats
- All foods containing food additives: artificial colors, flavors, preservatives, sweeteners, or texturing agents
- Frozen dinners, prepackaged meals
- All foods containing sugar or artificial sweeteners

RULE 3: CONSUME HEALTHY FATS

Healthy fats play an important role in fat metabolism and hormone production. In fact, eating too little fat can be disastrous and cause your body to hold on to trouble spot fat. Make a conscious effort to include in your diet healthy fats from sources such as cold-water fish, ground flaxseed, olive oil, and avocado. Also include foods such as:

Borage oil
Fish oil
Grapeseed oil
Olives
Organic heavy cream
Primrose oil
Raw almonds

For a complete list of healthy oils, refer to the food chart on page 117.

RULE 4: EAT MORE PROTEIN

Together with a calorie deficit, eating sufficient protein is absolutely critical for optimal body composition, immune function, metabolism, satiety, and performance. Protein helps replace worn-out cells, transports amino acids throughout the body, and aids in tissue growth and repair. If you are new to weight-training regimens such as those I provide in this book, I suggest you begin by consuming 0.8 grams of protein per pound of body weight each day. If this sounds like too much to handle, for the time being, simply focus on consuming a portion of protein every time you eat a meal.

RULE 5: DRINK MORE WATER

Water is pretty much a cure-all for many common health complaints, from arthritis to headaches. Proper hydration is also important for physical and mental performance and metabolism. The problems associated with chronic dehydration include increased appetite, weight gain, sore joints, and reduced cognitive and physical performance. Consume half your body weight in ounces each day (for example, a 120-pound woman should drink 60 ounces—about 8 cups—each day; a 200-pound man should drink 100 ounces—12 to 13 cups—each day), and more on days that you exercise or perspire heavily. You will have to pee more often than you are used to, so be sure to expect to take more bathroom breaks for the first week, until your body adjusts.

RULE 6: EAT MORE VEGGIES

Vegetables are fantastic to eat, as they contain lots of nutrients and very few calories. When you're trying to lose fat and improve your body composition, vegetables (the fibrous types, especially the leafy and green ones) should make up the bulk of your carbohydrate intake. Have a minimum of three servings of vegetables each day. If you prefer to have them all at once, that's okay.

The food chart on page 117 is a handy reference for which vegetables to incorporate into your diet. Some of my favorites are:

Arugula
Asparagus
Broccoli
Cabbage
Cauliflower
Celery
Collard greens
Cucumber
Green beans
Kale
Lettuce
Mushrooms
Peppers
Spinach

RULE 7: CUT BACK ON ALCOHOL

Alcohol is empty calories, and consumption of it often leads to poor food choices as well. You can have some alcohol, but you cannot consume it *ad libitum* and still expect to lose your trouble spot fat. I myself like the occasional drink, and I have discovered a trick to enjoying alcohol without gaining an ounce of fat. You will learn how you can do it too in chapter 5.

RULE 8: SUPPLEMENT YOUR DIET

Your body was designed to digest and assimilate whole foods; however, we don't always get everything we need from our diets, and supplements can help fill any gaps that may exist in your nutrient requirements. Subjecting your body to increased stress through physical training makes the need for supplements even greater. I discuss supplements in more detail later in the book, but for now, the four "foundational" supplements I recommend are:

1. Green food supplement, such as greens+
2. Fish oil
3. Multivitamin/multimineral
4. Vitamin D

RULE 9: KEEP A FOOD DIARY

One of the most underrated fat-loss tools is the food diary. The simple act of keeping track of what you eat and drink will bring awareness to your eating patterns and help you hold yourself accountable. I suggest keeping a food diary through-out the fat-loss process. Stats you should be monitoring include the type and approximate quantity of food and bever-age consumed, the time of day it's consumed, and any emo-tional triggers associated with it. Emotional triggers are those sounds, sights, smells, and situations that bring about a desire to eat or drink. These triggers can have a powerful impact on behavior and need to be identified in order to stop negative behaviors such as poor food choices and overconsumption from occurring on autopilot.

RULE 10: LIFT WEIGHTS

I discuss resistance (weight) training for trouble spots in greater detail in chapter 8 but, before we get there, begin train-ing your major muscle groups a minimum of two times per week. This training should include exercises such as squats, dead lifts, presses, lunges, and their many variations. If you are new to weight training, simply begin with Protocol 1 in chapter 8. If there is one rule of thumb to follow for resistance train-ing, it is this: *Always strive to increase your strength while maintain-ing proper form*. This maxim alone will have a significant impact on the amount of muscle your body will build. And no, you will not end up looking like a hulk or hulkette.

RULE 11: DO CARDIO

Cardiovascular exercise is an excellent way to burn calories and improve performance. You should be comfortable with performing one to two bouts of intense cardio exercise each week. Any more than that is unnecessary and can actually be detrimental. You will learn advanced cardio techniques for melting away trouble spot fat in chapter 8 as well.

RULE 12: MANAGE STRESS

Managing stress is a vital component to lasting health, long life, happiness, *and* fat loss. Recent studies show that approximately 40% of all North Americans suffer from adverse health effects due to stress. In addition, up to 90% of all visits to the doctor are for stress-related complaints or disorders. Stress has been linked to every leading cause of death, including cancer, heart disease, cirrhosis, accidental death, and suicide. At the same time, stress is a normal part of everyday life and can produce positive adaptations* if managed correctly. Effective stress-management techniques include meditation, deep breathing, and prayer.

RULE 13: SLEEP IT OFF

Get a minimum of seven to eight hours of sleep every night. Sleep in complete darkness (no night lights). A lack of sleep decreases the secretion of testosterone and human growth hormone (HGH), a hormone imperative for burning fat and building lean muscle tissue. Like testosterone, HGH also plays a role in controlling the body's fat and muscle proportions. It is

---

* "Adaptations" is a word you'll hear in fitness circles to refer to the changes, either positive or negative, in our bodies caused by our diet and exercise.

released in spurts during deep sleep. Too little sleep disrupts other hormones like *leptin*, which is responsible for telling your body when to eat. I discuss leptin in greater detail in chapter 4, but for now know that sleep debt causes leptin to decrease, resulting in cravings for fats and refined carbohydrates. Eating these foods in turn raises insulin levels, which add to fat gain. Sleeping in complete darkness triggers the pineal gland to release melatonin, which is a potent antioxidant that allows the body to regenerate while sleeping. Any light in the room (from a night light, clock radio, TV, etc.) will interfere with this process. Sleep in a cool room to aid in getting a restful night's sleep, too. Try passion flower extract if you experience trouble falling asleep, and time-released melatonin for help staying asleep. If you have trouble waking, simply dip your feet in cold water!

RULE 14: PRACTICE THE PARETO PRINCIPAL

Vilfredo Pareto was an economist best known for his observation in the early 1900s of wealth distribution. He noted that 80% of the wealth was held by 20% of the population. He then went on to show how this 80-20 relationship could be found everywhere, not just in economics. For example, Pareto explained that 80% of his garden peas were produced by 20% of the pea pods he had planted in his garden.

This rule applies to your diet and exercise too: as long as things are on track 80% of the time, whatever happens during the remaining 20% will have a negligible effect. In short, you don't have to live like a monk to get into great shape. You can eat more, train less, and still achieve dramatic, jaw-dropping results. Welcome to utopia, my friend!

Following these simple rules, especially the first, of eating fewer calories than you burn, will go a long way toward lowering your body fat percentage. Once you get to a level of 15%

body fat if you are a man and 20% if you are a woman, you will be looking pretty fit and will be left with only the trouble spot fat. And that you'll deal with by following the methods outlined in this book.

2

How to Get Your Ass in Gear
and Never Fail Again

I have a confession to make. I am often *very* lazy. I like to drink beer and eat pizza. My favorite pastime is watching a movie while doing both. I would have no problem retiring and doing just that.

So why don't I?

I will tell you why: fear. I am simply too scared of what would happen if I decided to give in to my delinquent urges.

Life coach Tony Robbins famously said that there are only two things motivating us to do all that we do: acquiring pleasure and avoiding pain. I disagree somewhat. I have seen many people lose sight of their goals even when there was a pleasurable reward waiting for them on the horizon. Back in the late 1990s, I worked with the sports-nutrition company EAS and the Body-for-LIFE Challenge. One of my responsibilities was to recruit participants for the challenge, which awarded prizes for the best 12-week body transformation. Business was booming, and thousands of people entered with hopes of winning the top prize, a brand-spanking-new Chevy Corvette. Yet despite having such a reward, only a very small percentage of participants completed the full 12-week program. Most folks abandoned ship after only a week or two, once they realized that transforming one's body isn't exactly a walk in the park. The possibility of a pleasurable (and valuable) reward wasn't enough for them to stay the course and follow through. Pleasure doesn't always work as a motivator. Pain avoidance, on the other hand, tends to work like a charm.

I use pain avoidance all the time to motivate me to get my butt in gear. Here is what I am afraid of.

FEAR OF REGRESSION

I have a picture that nobody else has ever seen. It is a picture that was taken of me standing shirtless on a beach during the summer of 1987.

I look like total crap. I have a gut, my arms resemble two Q-tips, and I have the muscle tone of a well-fed hippo. To top it all off, my haircut resembles the lead singer from A Flock of Seagulls (go to YouTube for a quick reminder).

Not exactly my proudest moment.

So, why on earth would I keep this photo? The answer is simple: I never want to look like that again. Ever.

Photographs are excellent reminders of what may happen if you stop taking care of your body. Humans have a tendency to romanticize the past, remembering all the good times and forgetting the bad. I want you to do the opposite. It is time to scare yourself half to death and give yourself a reminder of why you're cleaning up your act.

> **WORK WITH FEAR**
>
> Find a picture of what you don't want to look like (not neces-
> sarily of yourself) and put it where you will see it every day. I
> guarantee that doing so will leave you with a deeper motivation
> to change your habits and never go back.

FEAR OF LOSS

One of my favorite TV shows is *Till Debt Do Us Part*. The show is
about how couples can get into trouble financially if they don't
watch their spending. Host Gail Vaz-Oxlade does a fantastic job
of making people face the reality of their foolish ways. A light
always turns on inside the heads of the wayward couples when
they catch a glimpse of how much debt they will have in five
years' time if things don't change. Gail basically scares the shit
out of them and then shows them a way out. This is a great
strategy that works more often than not.

A recent study published in *Science* supports the notion that
people are incredibly loss averse. Researchers posed this scenario to subjects:

If you were given $50 and the following two choices, what
would you do?

- Keep $30.
- Gamble, with a 50-50 chance of keeping or losing the
  entire $50.

The researchers found that 43% of the subjects chose to
gamble. The options were then changed to:

- Lose $20.
- Gamble, with a 50-50 chance of keeping or losing the
  entire $50.

Some 62% of the subjects chose to gamble. What is interesting is that both dollar amounts are identical! Yet when the perceived risk of loss is higher, more people will choose to avoid that option.

You may be doing this already each year when you go to file your taxes. My accountant recently told me that his clients often say that they don't care so much about receiving a tax refund just so long as they don't have to pay more tax. They instruct him to play things safe and not be too aggressive in pursuing write-offs and refunds so as to avoid any scrutiny that may result in a financial penalty.

WORK WITH FEAR

Make a bet with a coworker or friend that you will reach your fitness goal by a predetermined time or pay a penalty. The rule of the bet is that if you fail to reach your objective, you must pay your coworker or friend $500. To make this even more motivating, make a bet with someone you really don't like. The thought of having to pay that person $500 simply because you couldn't stick to your diet and exercise routine is enough to keep most mortals on track.

FEAR OF EMBARRASSMENT

Most of us go to great lengths to avoid embarrassment.

Certainly, you don't want to be embarrassed in front of your colleagues, clients, or family. Employees don't want to be embarrassed in front of their coworkers or bosses. Business partners don't want to be embarrassed in front of their subordinates. This fear of embarrassment can help you lose body fat.

Recently, a TV program recruited volunteers for a weight-loss contest. They had to lose 15 pounds in two months or a picture of them in a bathing suit would be revealed on national television. The threat of public embarrassment worked, and all the participants were able to reach their weight-loss goals.

Fear of negative consequences drives this type of external motivation. Negative consequences influence behavioral changes to a greater extent than do positive consequences, and as a result, people will work harder to avoid pain than to receive pleasure.

WORK WITH FEAR

Take photographs of yourself in a bathing suit and hand them off to a trusted friend. Instruct your friend to post the pictures on the Internet if you fail to follow through on your body recomposition commitment.

TIME FOR ACTION

Before you read any further (and while the words of this chapter are still fresh in your mind), I would like to encourage you to take an important step.

Take a "before" picture. Put on a bathing suit and have a good friend take photos of you from the front, side, and rear. If you are too shy for that, do it yourself using a camera with a timer or a webcam. Make two copies of the photos. Post one of each on your bathroom mirror, refrigerator, and near your desk (or similar) at work. Take the other set of pictures and do as described in the "Fear of Embarrassment" section above, giving them to a friend to post on the Internet if you break your body recomposition commitment.

Your other option is to do nothing. This is what most people do—and then wonder why nothing ever changes in their lives. Don't be that person. Take action now.

PART TWO
THE SIMPLE SCIENCE OF FAT LOSS

3

The Skinny on Fat

Here is a quick exercise for you to do: Take off your clothes and stand in front of a mirror (please do this at home and not at the office). Take a look at your body and realize that yours is the most remarkable life form in existence. (This means all humans, so don't go getting a swelled head just yet.) Your body is the result of millions of years of evolution, and humans have experienced a lot over this vast expanse of time. We've learned to adapt to never-ending changes to our environment. Our bodies have one ultimate goal—survival—and we have developed many defenses to ensure that it happens.

Take a look at your body fat, for example. While you may not like how it looks or the impact it has on your wardrobe selection, your body fat does have a meaningful purpose. As stored energy, fat is your body's insurance policy against starvation. It wasn't that long ago that food was much harder to come by than it is today. Having extra fat meant that you would not starve to death if your next meal was a few weeks away instead of a few hours. Fat is actually very good at its job, as it provides a lot of stored energy without requiring much energy to sustain itself. Your fat cells can store an unlimited number of calories, and if they get full, they can multiply to allow even more calories to be stored. They are easy to create and quite difficult to get rid of. Your body loves them and couldn't care less that you don't. In short, losing those last pounds of body fat is not something your body really wants to do, but that does not mean it isn't possible—you just have to know how. Oh, and by the way, you can put your clothes back on now.

WHAT EXACTLY IS FAT, ANYWAY?

Fat, also known as *adipose tissue,* has several essential functions in the body. First, as mentioned above, it is a source of stored energy. One pound of fat is equal to approximately 3500 calories of ready-to-use energy. The average person has 30 pounds (or more) of body fat, which is over 100,000 calories of stored energy. This means that you could survive for over a month with nothing more than water and oxygen.

A second essential function of body fat is its cushioning action for the internal organs. An athlete—a linebacker playing football, say—is better off having some extra fat to protect him from the extreme physicality of the sport. For the rest of us, fat acts as an insulator, keeping us warm during periods of cold.

Body fat also plays a role in hormone production. According to a study published in the *Journal of Proteome Research*, fat is an active organ that sends chemical signals to other parts of the body. Rather than just sitting there and doing nothing, fat cells secrete certain hormones, much like other organs do. Among these hormones is leptin, which controls appetite, and *adiponectin*, which makes the body more sensitive to insulin, controls blood sugar levels, and helps speed up metabolism. Also, the hormones *DHEA* and *androstenedione* (both precursors to male and female sex hormones) are metabolized in the fat cells along with testosterone, which is converted to estrogen in males and postmenopausal women. Athletes need to be diligent about maintaining a low body fat percentage, since a higher percentage of body fat means more estrogen and less testosterone, and ultimately poorer performance.

Finally, body fat affects immune system function. The body fat reduction techniques described in this book will take you to body fat levels you never thought possible. I caution you, though, to use these techniques wisely. Staying at very low body fat levels for extended periods can negatively impact your immune system. Note, though, that having excessive amounts of body fat will have the same effect.

It would be wrong to believe that your body fat has no purpose other than to make you feel insecure in a bathing suit. The fact is that having some body fat is necessary for your health and survival. However, all fat cells are not created equal. When we think of fat we think of the stuff we can see, but there are actually a few different types of body fat.

VISCERAL FAT

Visceral fat is a type of body fat that exists in the abdomen and surrounds the internal organs. Everyone has some, especially those who are sedentary, chronically stressed, or maintain unhealthy diets. Visceral fat is different from subcutaneous fat (the visible fat that builds up under the skin) and has a very negative impact on health. In fact, excessive deposits of visceral fat are associated with many serious health problems, including cardiovascular disease, insulin resistance, and increased blood pressure. The one good thing about visceral fat is that it is quite easy to reduce, in part because it responds readily to exercise. In the hierarchy of fat loss, visceral fat tends to be the first type of fat that is lost when a person begins a healthy diet and exercise program.

BROWN FAT

Brown fat, or *brown adipose tissue* (BAT) fat, has garnered more attention as of late with the discovery that it has the ability to burn a significant number of fat calories from other fat sources in the body. In one study published in the *Journal of Clinical Investigation*, researchers discovered that stimulating BAT fat by exposing subjects to a cold environment increased metabolism by a whopping 80%! BAT fat produces a lot of heat. Its *thermogenic* (heat-producing) capacity is such that it allows mammals to live in cold, below-thermal-neutral conditions without having to rely on shivering muscles. Babies have more brown fat than adults do, and this is why they don't shiver when cold. As well, recent studies show that women tend to have more brown fat than men, with most of it located near the neck, chest, and upper back.

WHITE FAT

Compared with brown fat, white fat is far more abundant in the body. White fat develops rapidly with increased calorie intake, and its job is to store energy and produce hormones. White fat also tends to be lost quite easily (and evenly) when calories are reduced. Researchers recently discovered a new hormone called *irisin*, which converts white fat into the metabolically active brown fat discussed just above. This conversion occurs during exercise and is why the calories burned as a result of your workout exceed the number actually used in doing the activity itself. According to a study published in the *Nature International Weekly Journal of Science*, exercise training induces the expression of a gene in human muscle known as *FNDC5*, which produces irisin.

GOOSEBUMPS AND SHIVERS:
HOW TO ACTIVATE YOUR BROWN FAT

Exposure to mild cold stimulates brown fat energy expenditure. To induce your BAT to burn calories, you have to reduce your body temperature. Researchers reporting in the *New England Journal of Medicine* found that exposing both lean and overweight men to "mild cold exposure" (61°F/16°C) activated BAT in 23 out of 24 of them, whereas thermal-neutral temperatures resulted in zero BAT activity. The goal is to reduce body temperature to the point of goosebumps but not so far that you turn into a shivering mess. Here is how you can do it:

Method 1: Cold shower. Reduce the water temperature to below room temperature or less than 68°F (20°C) and stand with your upper back and neck facing the water stream. Remain under the cold water for at least five minutes. If at first this is too difficult, try alternating between warm (104°F/40°C) and cold (sub 68°F/20°C) water in 30-second intervals.

Method 2: Cold room. This technique is pretty simple: just turn down the heat. A study reported in the May 2010 issue of *Obesity* showed significant increases in BAT activity in about half of those who were kept for 2 hours in a 66°F (19°C) room, and no increase in BAT activity in those who were in an 80°F (27°C) room.

Method 3: Ice pack. Place an ice pack on your upper back for 20 to 30 minutes each day. This can be done while watching TV or working on the computer, for example.

Method 4: Ice bath. Fill the bathtub with cold water and ice cubes. Immerse yourself up to the waist for 10 minutes, three times per week. This is not for the faint of heart (literally).

Method 5: Ice water. Drink 2 cups of ice water three times per day. This is the least effective method for activating BAT, but it is also the easiest to do and can be performed anytime (as opposed to taking an ice bath, for example).

The hormone then changes white fat into brown fat, enhancing metabolism and hence caloric expenditure. This makes a very good case for accompanying diet with exercise to achieve optimal results.

Subcutaneous Fat

Subcutaneous fat is your body's most abundant form of white fat, making up approximately half of all fat in your body. This fat is located just beneath the skin and is generally the type of fat people are most interested in losing to look better. Losing significant amounts of subcutaneous fat is relatively simple with exercise and diet modifications.

Although subcutaneous fat can be found all over the bodies of both men and women, there are variations in distribution patterns between the sexes. Men have a tendency to carry more subcutaneous fat in their lower back and abdominal areas, resulting in an "android" or "apple" body shape. It is not uncommon for a man to have lean arms and legs while still carrying significant amounts of fat around the midsection. As his subcutaneous fat percentages increase, a man may find his chest also gaining fat. One thing is for certain: men rarely have fat thighs or calves. This seems to happen only once a man has reached the level of morbid obesity.

Most women's bodies, on the other hand, will happily store excess calories in subcutaneous fat cells surrounding the hips, thighs, and buttocks, resulting in a "gynoid" or "pear" body shape. As her subcutaneous fat percentages increase, a woman may find her belly, back, and arms also expanding. Unlike a man, fat thighs and calves are not uncommon on a woman, even if the rest of her body is relatively lean.

Trouble Spot Fat

Trouble spot fat is a type of subcutaneous fat that is resistant to typical dieting and exercising. Trouble spot fat is the last fat to leave your body and the first fat to return once your diet has ended. It is found in different locations depending on your sex.

For a man, trouble spot fat is almost always the last bits of fat that reside on the lower abdominals and lower back. This is the hardest fat for a man to lose and is what prevents most men from ever having a true six-pack. For a woman, trouble spot fat is more pervasive. As she loses fat, she will lose from her arms, upper back, abdominals, and lower back first (usually in that order). Last to leave will be the trouble spot fat that surrounds her hips, buttocks, and thighs.

Body fat distribution patterns differ greatly between the sexes, but as a general rule will reduce in the following order: visceral fat, subcutaneous fat, and, finally, trouble spot fat. To better understand why trouble spot fat is so difficult to lose, we need to examine how fat is burned by the body in the first place.

HOW YOUR BODY BURNS FAT

Fat cells are distinctly different from many other cells in the body and metabolically can do many different things. Fat cells can increase in number (*hyperplasia*) and in size (*hypertrophy*), and new fat cells can be formed (*lipogenesis*). These processes cause an *increase* in fat. In terms of *decreasing* fat, there are only two options: fat cells can break down and release their contents (*lipolysis*), or fat cells can die (*apoptosis*).

Apoptosis: How Your Fat Cells Are Killed

Let's begin by first focusing on apoptosis, or fat cell death. This is a great place to start: almost every client I have ever had has admitted to harboring homicidal thoughts toward their problem fat areas. Any person who has taken his or her body fat to low levels knows that fat cells are very resilient—once they have arrived, pretty much the only way to get rid of them is to surgically suck them out with a hose. Only by dieting down to near-starvation levels can we get fat cells to roll over and play dead. As this is obviously not a practical nor a healthy solution, we have to look to science for an alternative.

Recent research into fat cell death has provided some new hope for those of us who are interested in sending our fat cells into permanent retirement. In a German study, researchers looked into CLA (*conjugated linoleic acid*, a type of fat found mostly in meat and dairy products) and its impact on fat cell metabolism. The results were interesting. They concluded that CLA may actually *kill* your fat cells. The research continues, but it is well documented that CLA does aid in body fat reduction (either by lipolysis or apoptosis, but who really cares how so long as the end result is the same).

Many of the foods we eat daily contain CLA, including, as mentioned, beef and dairy products. Grass-fed cattle are a better source than are their grain-fed counterparts (and even then you would have to consume quite a lot in order to get a therapeutic dose of CLA). For this reason, I recommend taking a supplemental form at a dose of 3 to 6 grams per day.

CLA is not the only game in town. In another German study, researchers discovered that *resveratrol* (yes, the compound found in red wine) induces fat cell apoptosis too. Researchers found that this phytochemical, which is known for increasing lifespan and improving health, also contributes to fat cell death, stating that resveratrol "primed fat cells for apoptotic depletion." Call me crazy, but I have a sneaking suspicion that you like this news.

I wish there was more that could be said about permanently eliminating unwanted fat cells from your body, but unfortunately the research is simply not there yet. For the time being, we can try taking a CLA supplement and then focusing on the second (and most effective) way to lose body fat: lipolysis, the process in which fat cells break down and release their content.

Lipolysis: How Your Body "Loses" Fat

The first thing to understand is that your body does not actually lose fat. When conditions are right, fat cells release their stored contents, *triglycerides*. This means that the fat cell does not disappear. It only shrinks by releasing triglycerides, which are then burned by the body. That's right—the fat cells you created from your two-week Caribbean cruise with the all-you-can-eat buffets are with you for life. The only way to completely get rid of them is through liposuction or by apoptosis. But although we may not be able to get rid of them completely, we *can* shrink fat cells so that they no longer tick us off when we catch a glimpse of ourselves in the mirror.

The first step to shrinking your fat cells is to get the triglycerides out of them and to a place where they can be burned. To do this we must call on the action of the *catecholamines* (the hormones *adrenaline* and *noradrenaline*, otherwise known as *epinephrine* and *norepinephrine*) and an enzyme called *hormone-sensitive lipase*, or HSL.

According to "rogue nutritionist" Dr. Jonny Bowden, "HSL literally dissolves the stored fat that you have . . . into smaller components called fatty acids, which your body then burns for energy. HSL is what unlocks the doors to your fat cells." HSL is an adrenaline-sensitive, fat-metabolizing substance in fat tissue. (This point is important and will make sense in a moment.) Adrenaline, the catecholamine released by the sympathetic nervous system during exercise, binds to specific receptors on the fat cells, which in turn activates HSL. Lipolysis (fat breakdown) occurs as HSL breaks apart triglycerides held in the fat tissue and releases free fatty acids into the bloodstream.*

Once in the bloodstream, the free fatty acids are transported to the muscle cells and across the cell membranes to the *mitochondria* (the structures responsible for energy production within a cell), where they are oxidized or "burned." The number of free fatty acid transporters on the muscle cell membrane can increase with exercise, enhancing the body's ability to metabolize fat.

If the catecholamines are the hormones that turn on HSL release, then insulin is the hormone that shuts it off. The presence of even small amounts of insulin in the bloodstream is enough to inactivate HSL and shut down fat burning. This effect is more pronounced in individuals who have less workout experience, as they utilize insulin less efficiently compared with those who are more highly trained.

There is another key hormone involved in lipolysis: *cyclic adenosine monophosphate*, or cAMP. This is a messenger that reacts with the catecholamine hormones to direct changes within the cells. Fat mobilization can occur only when cAMP is high. Catecholamines increase cAMP, and insulin reduces it.

Clearly, the catecholamines are important when it comes to fat burning. They are a double-edged sword, though, as they can send different signals to your body, depending on which receptors they interact with. All over the various tissues of your body (including fat tissue) are cells called *adrenoceptors*, which react in response to the messages sent by the catecholamines. Among the adrenoceptors are two main classes, alpha and beta. The functions of alpha receptors include inhibiting lipolysis and blood flow to fat tissues. Beta receptors, on the other hand,

---

* High-intensity interval training (HIIT) is the ideal way to increase the release of the catecholamine hormones. HIIT is explained in greater detail in chapter 8.

increase lipolysis and blood flow to fat tissues.When the cate-cholamines interact with beta receptors, cAMP is amplified and fat burning is increased. Conversely, when the catecholamines interact with alpha receptors, cAMP is reduced and fat burning is decreased. Obviously, it would be preferable to have more beta receptors (and fewer alpha receptors) to assist in fat burn-ing. Unfortunately, the ratio of alpha receptors to beta recep-tors varies significantly in different parts of the body. According to researcher Lyle McDonald, "Lower body fat (hips and thighs) has been found to have roughly nine times as many alpha receptors as beta receptors." Trouble spot fat will always have a greater density of alpha receptors than beta. The reverse is also true—fat deposits that are the easiest to lose have a greater density of beta receptors than alpha.

And herein lies a key message of this book, the reason fat is so troublesome and why men and women have different fat patterns: women have more alpha and fewer beta receptors in fat cells surrounding their stomachs, hips, and thighs, and men have more alpha and fewer beta receptors in fat cells surround-ing their chests, bellies, and love handle areas.

The best way to lose fat in these areas is to activate the beta receptors while simultaneously blocking the alpha receptors. This can be accomplished in two ways:

1. **Follow a low-carb diet.** Diets that are low in carbo-hydrates (less than 20% of total calories) will reduce insulin, inhibit alpha receptors, and increase the release of the catecholamine hormones. This effect does not happen immediately. Carbs must be reduced for several days for the full effect to occur. According to research, short-term fasting of 14 to 20 hours will have the same effect.

2. **Perform high-intensity exercise.** Even moderate exercise will increase catecholamine output and activate

beta receptors; however, high-intensity exercise is significantly more effective. That being said, high-intensity exercise *alone* is not sufficient for removing trouble spot fat. Although high-intensity exercise is great for releasing fat into the bloodstream, if its duration is too short, fat that is not burned will *re-esterify*—in other words, get stored again. This problem can be solved by extending the duration of the exercise session to allow for the released fatty acids to be burned rather than restored. Combining high- and moderate-intensity exercise within the same workout in order to extend its length accomplishes this.

As discussed, when the catecholamines react with beta receptors in a fat cell, fatty acids are released into the bloodstream, where they can be transported to muscle tissues to be burned. An increase in the efficiency of blood flow to fat cells amplifies this effect by boosting the interaction between adrenaline and fat-tissue beta receptors. Poor blood flow means adrenaline can't reach the fat cells, making it harder to mobilize fat away from the cell. When compared with other fat deposits, areas where fat is very difficult to lose tend to be denser and cooler to the touch, which is associated with poorer blood flow (cellulite is an excellent example of this). Increasing blood flow can be accomplished in two ways:

1. **Increased exercise.** Vigorous exercise is one of the best ways to increase blood flow and the transportation of fat to muscle cells, where it can be burned. But this process is amplified in the presence of low levels of *glycogen* in the muscle (glycogen is a combination of sugar and water that is stored in your muscles and liver). The exercise programs detailed in this book are excellent

for depleting glycogen and promoting more blood flow through fat tissue.

2. **Short-term fasting.** In terms of nutrition, short-term fasting also improves blood flow to fat cells, moving fat to your muscles, where it can be burned as fuel.

A NOTE ON SPOT REDUCTION

In a 2007 study published in the *American Journal of Physiology*, researchers tested male subjects after an overnight fast and discovered that blood flow and fat burning are increased in subcutaneous fat tissue adjacent to contracting muscles. Researchers concluded that if you were to vigorously train one muscle or localized group of muscles, blood flow to the fat surrounding that area would be increased, *potentially* increasing the mobilization of fatty acids from that area. In other words, spot reduction may not be a myth after all. But before you drop this book and start performing hundreds of stomach crunches, listen up: any good body-transformation coach will tell you that it's not that simple. The fundamental rules of fat loss still apply, and you still have to induce a calorie deficit in order to lose trouble spot fat. Nevertheless, what we can learn from this study is that if you have a trouble spot, it would be wise to train the muscles surrounding the area and to do so when insulin levels are very low—for example, in a fasted state.

It's important to know what body fat is and the different types you have in your body. Understanding the mechanisms behind fat breakdown and mobilization, and why men and women have different fat patterns, will arm you with the information you need as you embark on the Trouble Spot Fat Loss program. Perhaps of greatest importance is your newfound understanding of the catecholamine hormones and adrenoceptor function, and how these can be affected by diet and exercise.

Let's now examine the body's master messengers, which are in control of the entire fat-burning and muscle-building process—your hormones.

4

Trouble Spot Fat and Hormones

Various hormones in your body can affect the type of fuel you burn (fat or sugar) and from where on your body the fat is taken (stomach, hips, thighs, etc.). If you are serious about dropping pounds of fat from your trouble spots, you need to pay attention, as these 11 hormones are crucial to fat mobilization and burning. For certain hormones, for example testosterone and estrogen, I have included levels to be used as an index of the healthy range of these hormones in the body. I recommend seeing your healthcare provider to get your levels tested.

THE CATECHOLAMINES: ADRENALINE AND NORADRENALINE

Adrenaline and noradrenaline are the catecholamine hormones that travel through the blood and message your adrenoceptor cells to mobilize fat for fuel. The catecholamines will also increase blood pressure, heart rate, and the need to urinate, while simultaneously decreasing appetite. If the catecholamines are released in the presence of high leptin or insulin (discussed in the coming pages), the body will burn sugar preferentially over fat. But when you eat a low-carbohydrate diet for an extended period, you increase catecholamine release and begin burning fat instead of sugar. Any stresses will increase production of these hormones, but the best (and healthiest) way for you to release adrenaline is through high-intensity exercise. I cannot overstate the importance of exercise in a fat-loss program. Caffeine will also increase catecholamine release by a small amount (good news for us java lovers). Just keep it black and organic, with no added sugar. Fat-burning supplements containing ephedrine or synephrine will increase catecholamine release too.

CORTISOL

Although often demonized, cortisol is good or bad depending on the situation. If cortisol is released in the presence of high insulin, low testosterone, and low human growth hormone (HGH), it acts as a fat-storing, muscle-burning hormone. If released in the presence of low insulin, high testosterone, and high HGH, it enhances fat burning and muscle preservation. Despite what you may have seen on late-night TV, cortisol should not be blocked in the body. Rather, it needs to be kept in balance. If you were to eliminate cortisol, it would not be available to drive free fatty acids into the muscle cells, which would cause your adrenal glands to work overtime, leading to adrenal fatigue, weak muscles, loss of appetite, and hypoglycemia.

Cortisol is a *glucocorticoid*, meaning that it has the ability to increase blood glucose levels. This occurs as part of the fight-or-flight response, when cortisol assumes control of the body's metabolic systems during high-stress events, temporarily increasing the flow of glucose (as well as of protein and fat) out of your tissues and into the bloodstream. This increases physical readiness and energy so that you are able to handle the stressful situation. However, when stress is prolonged through excessive worry, overwork, inadequate sleep, disease, overtraining, or poor nutrition, cortisol's temporary job becomes a permanent one, and this taxes your adrenals, leading to adrenal fatigue and low cortisol (also not good). This condition is not uncommon; symptoms include joint pain, cravings for sweet and salty foods, excessive thirst, and even lower back pain. The only way to know for sure if your cortisol is off-kilter is through testing by your physician or natural-health-care provider. Here are nine steps to keep cortisol in balance.

1. **Avoid very-low-calorie diets**, especially for periods longer than 14 days. The chronic restriction of calories is a significant stress to the body, causing decreases in testosterone and increases in cortisol.

2. **Avoid overtraining** (a common mistake among overzealous newbies). Keep workouts brief (less than 60 minutes) and intense by packing more work into less time.

3. **Consume protein immediately following your workout.** This will help maximize recovery.

4. **Be sure to get seven to eight hours of deep, restful sleep nightly in a dark room.**

5. **Drink plenty of water.**

6. **Do not binge on alcohol.**

7. **Eat a healthy diet.** Consume an alkalinizing, healthy diet rich in essential fatty acids, green vegetables, and protein, and low in processed foods and sugar.

8. **Increase supplementation** of vitamin C (minimum 2 grams daily), and use an adrenal support supplement.

9. **Have your DHEA levels tested** and supplement if
   necessary. DHEA is a steroid hormone secreted by the
   adrenal glands, and when levels drop too low, your
   endocrine function will be compromised. Low DHEA
   levels may also be a sign of stressed adrenals. The only
   way to know if you have low DHEA is through testing.
   Ask your doctor to run an "adrenal panel" and review
   the results with you.

GHRELIN

Ghrelin is a hormone produced in the stomach that serves to
signal hunger and causes your stomach to growl. It is the only
known appetite stimulant made outside the brain. Ghrelin
levels increase before eating and decrease afterward. In a study
published in *ScienceDaily*, researchers discovered that ghrelin
not only stimulates the brain, giving rise to an increase in appetite, but also favors the accumulation of visceral fatty tissue,
which surrounds internal organs and is considered to be the
most harmful type of fatty tissue.

Ghrelin is a "psychic" hormone in that its levels will
increase in anticipation of a meal. Ghrelin levels are controlled primarily by food intake and will increase while fasting. Ghrelin is reduced by eating, especially carbohydrates and
proteins, as these lessen its production and release to a greater
extent than fats.

Ghrelin appears to have a sort of "set point" that is determined by meal patterns. The more you restrict your calories, the
lower the set point for ghrelin. Ghrelin levels tend to decrease
naturally after you fast for a few days, which means that after
fasting for more than 48 hours, your hunger diminishes.

By decreasing meal frequency and caloric intake for as little
as a few days, you can lower the attendant cravings. This is
an important point to remember if you find yourself gaining

weight—fast for 24 hours and you will become less hungry and regain some control.

INSULIN

Depending on where you go for health and fitness information, you have probably heard drastically different things about the hormone insulin. On one hand are those who say insulin is the root cause of obesity and needs to be kept under control at all times. On the other hand are professional bodybuilders who inject insulin so as to increase fat loss and muscle size. So, is insulin good or bad?

The truth is, it depends. But before we continue, first, a brief overview of insulin.

Insulin regulates the levels of sugar in your blood. When you eat a meal, the carbohydrates in the meal are broken down into *glucose* (a sugar used as energy by your cells). The glucose then enters your blood, and your pancreas senses the rising glucose and releases insulin. Insulin allows the glucose to enter the cells of your liver, muscles, and fat. Once your blood glucose starts to come back down, insulin levels come back down too. This cycle happens all day, every day. You eat a meal, glucose goes up and insulin goes up. After a short while, glucose goes back down, and insulin goes down too. Insulin levels are directly related to food intake and are typically lowest in the early morning, since it's usually been at least seven to eight hours since your last meal.

Regulating blood sugar isn't insulin's only job. For example, it stimulates muscle to build more protein through a process known as *protein synthesis*. It also inhibits the breakdown of fat (lipolysis) and stimulates the creation of fat (lipogenesis). The truth is, we need insulin, and it is perfectly healthy for insulin to rise and fall in conjunction with our meal patterns. The vilification of insulin in many diet books has caused people to hold many false beliefs about it. Here are a few of the common ones:

Myth: I can eat as much as I want and still lose weight so long as I don't eat carbohydrates and spike insulin.

Truth: To lose weight, you can eat as much as you want (carbohydrates, fats, or proteins) so long as you remain in a calorie deficit. There is no evidence to support otherwise and never will be.

Myth: Only carbohydrates spike insulin.

Truth: Protein also raises insulin, in some cases surpassing the insulin response to white bread (as happens with whey protein). One study found beef to stimulate just as much insulin secretion as brown rice. The fact is that protein is a potent stimulator of insulin secretion, and this insulin secretion is not related to changes in blood sugar or glucose creation from the protein. This indicates that there is a lot more behind insulin secretion than just carbohydrate consumption.

Without having to be converted to glucose first, the amino acids (the building blocks of protein) directly stimulate your pancreas to produce insulin. This is an important distinction, as a rise in insulin is not necessarily an indication of high blood glucose.

Insulin *does not* have to be kept as low as possible at all times in order to lose fat. But we don't want high insulin levels on a continual basis. In a healthy individual, high insulin levels are typically cleared within 10 minutes. This is not so with individuals who have poor glucose tolerance. The problem is that many of the foods that produce high insulin levels (such as refined-wheat products and sugar-filled beverages) stimulate appetite and do not promote satiety, causing people to eat more calories and gain weight.

The bottom line is that insulin isn't the cause of your trouble spot fat. It is better to focus on improving how well your cells respond to insulin by eating a diet rich in healthy proteins, fiber, fats, and vegetables, and by eliminating processed foods, rather than focusing on keeping insulin as low as possible every second of the day.

Myth: Foods that produce high levels of insulin make you fat.

Truth: Although insulin will suppress the actions of hormone-sensitive lipase (HSL, the substance that helps break apart fat deposits), so will high fat intake. Regardless of whether you follow the Zone Diet, the Atkins Diet, or the government's national food guide, you still have to watch how much food you eat and be in a calorie deficit in order to lose fat. It is perfectly fine for insulin levels to rise and fall periodically throughout the day (as they do every time you eat). Problems arise when blood sugar levels remain elevated over an extended period because of poor insulin management or insulin resistance.

GLUCAGON

Glucagon functions similarly to insulin as it breaks down stored glycogen (a combination of sugar and water) in the liver and releases sugars for energy. The difference between glucagon and insulin is that insulin lowers your blood glucose by helping your body use the glucose in the blood for energy. Glucagon raises your blood glucose by causing the liver and muscles to release stored glucose quickly.

Injectable glucagon is used by people with type 1 diabetes when experiencing a low-blood-sugar emergency. Although glucagon was once believed to help with fat burning, this has been proven to be false. It may not help with the burning of body fat per se, but it does work to increase satiety. After a protein-rich meal, your body releases glucagon to counterbalance insulin and reduce appetite.

ADIPONECTIN

Adiponectin is a hormone produced in fat cells. Adiponectin increases the use of fatty acids for fuel while enhancing insulin sensitivity and reducing inflammation in your circulatory system. If you have adequate levels of adiponectin, you will likely have a healthy range of insulin production, improved blood sugar management, and a much easier time controlling your weight.

However, if your weight increases, adiponectin production is reduced. In healthy individuals, leptin and adiponectin levels rise and fall together, but when a person gains fat, leptin rises and adiponectin falls, increasing the risk of insulin resistance, excess weight gain, type 2 diabetes, and cardiovascular inflammation.

Raising adiponectin levels is relatively simple and can be achieved by increasing your intake of omega-3 fatty acids and fibrous vegetables. The Anytime Meals recipes found on pages 229–241 are perfect for maintaining optimal levels of this important hormone.

LEPTIN

Derived from the Greek word *leptos*, "leptin" translates as "thin," and this hormone is one of the most important hormones when it comes to controlling hunger and losing body fat. Leptin, like adiponectin, is produced primarily in the fat cells, and its main function is to protect your body from starvation. Here is how your body sees things: the less body fat you have, the more food you need. Conversely, the more body fat you have, the less food required.

When leptin levels are high, you feel less hungry. Its levels scale with body fat percentage—the more fat you have, the more leptin you produce. However, someone with good leptin sensitivity will tend to stay naturally lean and not gain weight easily. Women typically produce two to three times more leptin than do men, but, during dieting, leptin levels drop much faster in women. This may explain why women have a harder time losing fat than men.

When you go through a period of calorie restriction (which is required to lose fat), leptin levels fall precipitously, and rebound very quickly when calories are dramatically increased. When leptin is low, feelings of hunger are relentless.* A decrease in leptin can also lower immune system function. This may be why people are more susceptible to colds and flus during extended periods of dieting.

In a nutshell, the amount of leptin your body produces is a direct reflection of the amount of body fat you carry and how much you eat. Remember too that your body perceives stored body fat as an energy reserve, not as a detriment to your aesthetic ideal. I am sure you have noticed with your own body how it is very easy to gain fat and much harder to lose it. This just plain sucks, I know, but it is the case for the vast majority of human beings. There is a simple evolutionary reason for this: as humans evolved, there was a risk of being too lean, and having extra pounds meant you could survive longer during periods when no food was available.

Your body doesn't worry about losing those last few pounds that are driving you crazy, and in fact wants to hold on to them as a means of survival should a famine occur. Leptin helps your body to do this by increasing hunger and decreasing metabolism as calories decrease.

---

* Leptin isn't the only hormone that decreases with calorie restriction. Levels of human growth hormone, thyroid, and testosterone also fall as your body slows its metabolism in response to the decrease in energy intake.

How to Increase Leptin

For a person following a low-calorie diet for an extended period, the answer to how to increase leptin is quite simple (and enjoyable): eat more. Pretty much all the negative adaptations that happen when you diet for a prolonged period can be reversed with a good old-fashioned cheat meal (or two).

I want to be clear on something: you *must* have been following a low-calorie/low-carb diet for several days (4 to 6 days minimum for men, 13 for women) in order for the cheat meal to work to your benefit. One day of dieting isn't enough—your body does not react that fast. There need to be several days of dieting (together with exercise) for leptin levels to drop.

Leptin Resistance

Leptin levels can decrease with dieting by as much as 50% in one week's time. This is one of the reasons very-low-calorie diets should never be followed for an extended period. But there is another issue that can impact leptin: leptin resistance.

As with insulin, your body can become resistant to the action of leptin. This is generally caused by years of having high body fat levels and eating a diet too high in processed foods. The condition is exacerbated by a high-fat, high-fructose diet.

Leptin resistance occurs when your body no longer utilizes leptin efficiently, even when high levels of the hormone are present. At this point, leptin can no longer do its job properly and won't help curb your appetite, losing much of its fat-loss benefits. People who develop leptin resistance have a very difficult time losing body fat and maintaining a healthy weight. This is commonly seen in overweight people who cannot control their appetite and food intake.

Preventing Leptin Resistance

Here are five ways that you can maintain adequate levels of leptin without growing resistant to its effects:

1. **Cut back on fructose.** Excess fructose increases blood triglycerides that block the passage of leptin to the brain. Consuming small amounts of berries is fine, but stay away from *gorging* on bananas, apples, peaches, and so on.

2. **Reduce intake of grains.** I always recommend that people start any diet by eliminating high-allergen foods such as dairy and wheat. One reason is that grains such as wheat, rye, and barley contain *lectins*, proteins that can bind to the leptin receptors and cause leptin resistance.

3. **Ensure adequate rest.** Being sleep deprived has been linked to lowered leptin levels. Be sure to get at least seven hours of restful sleep each night.

4. **Eat sufficient protein.** People who struggle to lose fat will always benefit from an increase in dietary protein. I have found that eating sufficient amounts of protein (together with healthy fats) for breakfast blunts hunger for many hours and provides excellent energy and focus. Leptin sensitivity will improve simply by substituting the typical North American breakfast staples (such as breakfast cereals and breads) for meat, eggs, nuts, and other protein foods. People who are leptin resistant should aim to consume 50 grams of protein at breakfast alone.

5. **Take regular diet breaks.** As discussed, consuming minimal calories for too long will reduce leptin levels and send hunger soaring and fat-burning hormones plummeting. To prevent this from happening,

I recommend scheduling in "refeed" days, when you increase your calorie and carbohydrate intake, weekly for men and every two weeks for women. But it is also important to not have extended periods of high-calorie days, as leptin resistance can occur quickly, making it very difficult to reduce calories back to normal intake. Many people experience this effect over the holidays, when high-calorie eating is often a daily event. Once the holiday feeding frenzy is over, they find it extremely hard to resume lower-calorie eating patterns and continue to gain weight.

One of the biggest problems a person faces when following a diet is the drop in leptin that happens as calories are reduced. Injecting leptin may solve this problem but is cost-prohibitive and unnecessary. The goal is not to raise leptin levels above baseline but rather to reverse or prevent the drop in leptin that otherwise will inevitably occur. When following a reduced-calorie diet, this goal can easily be achieved by having a "cheat" meal or two. When done correctly, this type of cyclical dieting is a powerful fat-loss technique, explained in detail in chapter 7.

TESTOSTERONE

Testosterone is widely known as the male hormone, though females have some too, but in much smaller amounts. In males, the Leydig cells in the testes produce testosterone, whereas in females the ovaries and adrenal glands perform this function, though to a much smaller extent.

Like other hormones in the body, testosterone is regulated by a feedback loop. If the body thinks there's too much, it reduces production or converts the excess into something else, such as the hormones *estradiol* (a form of estrogen) or *DHT* (*dihydrotestosterone*). This commonly happens in young males with normal testosterone levels who start using steroids in the pursuit of faster muscle gains. The conversion of excess testosterone then leads to problems such as gynecomastia (affectionately known as "bitch tits"), as well as hair loss—hardly the studly result a young man is trying to achieve.

Low testosterone levels are linked to a whole host of problems, including low sex drive, low sperm count, poor memory, and, of course, decreased muscle mass. On the other hand, individuals with levels that are on the high end of the normal range enjoy decreased incidence of heart disease, increased lifespan, and better mood, sex drive, memory and quality of life.

Normal serum total testosterone levels vary from person to person over time and generally decrease with age. On average, a healthy adult male will have testosterone levels ranging from 270 to 1070 ng/dL (9 to 38 nmol/L), while a healthy adult female's levels will range from 15 to 70 ng/dL (0.52 to 2.40 nmol/L).

Several factors can suppress testosterone output. These include:

- Chronically low-calorie intake for extended periods (more than 20% below basic maintenance needs for more than 14 days)
- Chronically high-calorie intake for extended periods
- A diet low in essential nutrients, resulting in vitamin and mineral deficiency
- A diet too low in fat
- A diet high in sugar or fructose (In addition to reducing testosterone, high sugar intake will decrease nitric oxide production. Nitric oxide dilates blood vessels. It is the same substance Viagra works to *increase*. Think about that the next time you have some soda while out on a big date.)

- Chronic depression
- Overuse of hormonal contraception
- Recreational drug use (chronic marijuana abuse will lower testosterone)
- Excessive alcohol consumption
- Overtraining
- Chronic stress and anxiety
- Being obese
- Persistent ill health
- Poor sleep
- Head injuries (concussion or any hard blow to the head can disrupt hormone production)

There may be another possible explanation for males suffering from low testosterone: cell phone radiation. In a study published in the *Saudi Medical Journal,* researchers exposed rats to radio frequency electromagnetic radiation from a mobile phone for one hour a day for 28 days. The results were shocking. In less than one month, the testosterone levels of the rats exposed to cell phone radiation had reduced significantly in comparison with the control group. Not only was testosterone lowered but so was sperm count, motility, and viability. Given all the problems surrounding fertility these days, it seems plausible that the rise of mobile phones may be partly to blame. These findings have prompted me to become diligent about shutting my phone down when it is on my hip and only turning it on periodically to check for messages.

Testosterone Determines Fat Patterning

The differences in fat patterning in men and women become evident as changes to testosterone levels occur. As a man's testosterone drops he can see a shift away from visceral fat toward hip, thigh, and chest fat, whereas when a woman enters menopause and experiences lower levels of the hormone, her hip, thigh, and chest fat will move toward visceral. Other symptoms of low testosterone (or "low T," as it is commonly known) include:

- Loss of lean body mass, including muscle and bone density, along with an increase in body fat
- Low sexual desire and sexual response (including difficulty achieving orgasm)
- Reduced strength
- High blood pressure
- Depression, mood swings, and loss of interest in everyday activities
- Blood test results that show a poor blood lipid profile for cholesterol and triglyceride levels

Low testosterone is a problem that can impede the loss of trouble spot fat and reduce the chances of achieving optimal body composition. If you suspect that you have low T, the first step is to see your primary care provider and request testing. Do not rely on anecdotal testing methods. You have to know what your numbers are and then track those numbers to observe any changes.

Endocrinologists are now starting to prescribe testosterone therapeutically, either for replacement (for example, in older men and women) or to treat symptoms of disease. This doesn't always solve the problem. Sometimes a person can have normal or even high levels of testosterone and still suffer from symptoms associated with low T. This happens when testosterone gets "bound" by *sex hormone binding globulin* (*SHBG*), effectively rendering it inert. SHBG can be increased in the body by a blood sugar imbalance, including a cortisol-induced blood sugar imbalance caused by stress. Other possible causes of poor testosterone usage include:

- Impaired liver detoxification function (the liver isn't filtering estrogen properly)
- Poor gastrointestinal health (in particular, low stomach acid, leading to dietary deficiencies)
- Altered adrenal function
- Impaired enzyme activity (such as impaired aromatase and 5-alpha reductase)
- Compromised pituitary function

A good naturopath can help assess your unique needs and may be able to correct any issue you have without having to resort to using synthetic testosterone. In this book, we are going to focus on optimizing the body's natural production of testosterone (and avoiding crashes) through intelligent training and nutrition strategies.

Strategies for Raising Testosterone Naturally

The diet and exercise methods outlined in this book are designed to optimize your body's anabolic hormone levels, including testosterone. In a nutshell, these strategies include:

- Lifting heavier weights and reducing your rest periods between sets
- Getting enough antioxidants and vitamin D
- Ensuring sufficient vitamin and mineral status, including that of zinc and calcium (which has been shown to increase testosterone levels)
- Eating healthy fats daily
- Hitting your daily protein requirements
- Getting enough sleep

One testosterone booster that is not well known is caffeine. Research has shown that having caffeine prior to training can increase testosterone levels by as much as 20%. But caffeine also raises cortisol, and this is why it should be used only before exercise.

ESTROGEN

No discussion on testosterone is complete without a discussion on estrogen. Recently, estrogen has been receiving some very bad press. Estrogen makes you fat, estrogen makes you crazy, estrogen is responsible for failed relationships. Of course, these statements are not entirely correct.

Known as the female sex hormone, estrogen is actually found in both men and women (men just have less, hopefully). In premenopausal women, the most important producer of estrogens is the ovaries. After menopause, things change as the ovaries gradually cease production of estrogen. At this time, fat tissue increases and becomes the new source of estrogen for a woman.

It's important to remember that excess body fat can disrupt proper hormonal balance—in both sexes. In men, the main source of estrogen is testosterone that has been converted. This process occurs in the fat cells of both sexes and presents a compelling reason to maintain a healthy body weight at all times.

Estrogen comes in three forms: *estradiol* (the most potent estrogen, produced by the ovaries), *estriol* (produced by the placenta during pregnancy), and *estrone* (the most dominant estrogen in menopausal women, produced by both the ovaries and fat tissue). But when we talk about estrogen we are usually talking about estradiol. Estriol and estrone each have about one-tenth the potency of estradiol.

If you want to compare them with your own blood work, normal levels of estradiol are as follows:

Males: less than 50 pg/ml

Females: follicular phase, 10 to 200 pg/ml; mid-cycle, 100 to 400 pg/ml; luteal phase, 15 to 260 pg/ml; and in postmeno-pausal women, less than 50 pg/ml

Estrogen imbalance, whether levels are too high or too low, can lead to various problems for both sexes, including an increased number of alpha receptors, decreased levels of cAMP (an important hormone for burning fat), and as a result, increased body fat. The following are steps that you can take to maintain a healthy estrogen balance:

1. **Digest your food properly.** You are not only what you eat—you are what you eat, digest, and assimilate. It is important that the nutrients you ingest are being properly absorbed. Foods that are cooked or processed often lack important enzymes that can impact how your body is using nutrients. Assuming that these are the types of food you consume, I recommend taking digestive enzymes with all your meals. Look for a digestive enzyme supplement that also contains hydrochloric acid (HCl). Most people have very low HCl levels, but it is required in order for foods to be properly assimilated into the body.

2. **Eat your veggies.** Vegetables such as broccoli, Brussels sprouts, cabbage, cauliflower, kale, and spinach can help your body eliminate bad estrogens. Broccoli is my personal favorite, as it contains indoles, which are known to help fight cancer and improve the liver's ability to rid the body of excess estrogen. The best way to maintain your broccoli's nutrient content is to cook it lightly steamed to crisp-tender, not boiled to mush as this reduces nutrient

content. I also recommend you choose organic whenever possible.

3. **Eat more wasabi.** Authentic wasabi root (not the green-colored horseradish that is often used as a substitute at cheap sushi restaurants) contains *Diindolylmethane,* or DIM. DIM is the active form of indole-3-carbinol, a compound found in cruciferous vegetables. DIM helps prevent the conversion of testosterone into estrogens.

4. **Take your supplements.** Fish oil, B vitamins, magnesium, and zinc can help your body properly metabolize estrogen.

5. **Drink filtered water.** A good-quality water filtration system can help minimize the amount of estrogen you are being exposed to through the water you drink. Consider a filter for your shower as well, as estrogen can be absorbed through the skin also.

6. **Consider your form of birth control.** Birth control pills will have an effect on female estrogen levels. An alternative form may be a better choice.

7. **Drink less booze.** Excessive alcohol consumption (especially of beer) will reduce testosterone and increase estrogen.

8. **Lift more weights.** Swap two (or more) days of cardio for resistance training. Lifting weights has a positive impact on your testosterone, HGH, and estrogen levels, whereas excessive cardio will have the opposite effect.

9. **Eat flaxseed.** According to expert trainer Charles Poliquin, when estrogen is bound to sex hormone binding globulin (SHBG), it's not available to bind with cellular receptors and therefore won't have its negative estrogenic impact. Poliquin says that

flaxseed hulls are especially effective at increasing SHBG.*

10. **Minimize exposure to xenoestrogens.** Xenoestrogens are environmental estrogens that can disrupt cellular metabolism and increase body fat. Sources include bisphenol A (found in plastic bottles and the lining of cans); phthalates (found in shower curtains, air fresheners, vinyl flooring, and shrink-wrap); PFOA, or C8 (found in Teflon, pizza boxes, and microwave popcorn bags); Gore-Tex (found in waterproof clothing); and various soy products. Xenoestrogens are also believed to be linked to hormonal disruption, resulting in sexual deformities in baby boys and reduced fertility in adult males.

Estrogen alone is not the cause of excess body fat in women. This is easy to prove if we simply look at menopausal women who gain body fat when estrogen goes *down*. If high estrogen levels were the cause of female trouble spot fat, then when estrogen goes down, so should fat. Some research even suggests that estrogen may actually aid in the mobilization of fatty acids from fat tissue because of its ability to enhance adrenaline and human growth hormone production, as well as increase the production of nitric oxide, that important molecule produced by the body that helps dilate blood vessels and improve blood flow (think Viagra).

I recommend that women work with their primary care provider to keep their estrogen levels in a healthy range. Both sexes will benefit by following the 10 steps listed above.

---

* Both high and low SHBG levels can create problems with sex hormone balance. Low SHBG levels are associated with other disorders too, including obesity, insulin resistance, and chronic high blood pressure. SHBG in high levels binds testosterone, preventing it from exerting its effects and increasing estrogen's impact.

HUMAN GROWTH HORMONE

Often touted as being the "fountain of youth," human growth hormone has a powerful effect on body composition. Secreted by the pituitary gland, HGH helps muscle, bone, and other tissues to grow, while preventing tissue breakdown (catabolism). HGH is also involved in the fat-burning process, although, compared with insulin and the catecholamines, it plays a secondary role.

Released from the anterior pituitary gland in short "spurts," HGH has a healthy reference range of 0.06 to 8.00 ng/ml. This release of HGH happens throughout the entire day, with the largest amount being released during sleep.

For someone who is HGH deficient, HGH replacement may be necessary; this condition must be diagnosed and monitored by a physician. HGH therapy is also extremely expensive, costing between $10,000 and $30,000 per year! This is obviously cost-prohibitive for most people, and unless you have a pituitary deficiency, completely unnecessary. Several lifestyle modifications that can help optimize your body's natural production of HGH are within your control.

Exercise and HGH

When done correctly, exercise can be a potent stimulator of HGH. Depending on the training methods and variables used, both cardiovascular training and resistance work can enhance HGH levels.

Cardiovascular Training

Although cardiovascular training is not normally associated with HGH release, recent research has shown that there is a link. Here are two ways in which you can increase HGH output using cardiovascular training:

1. **Incorporate interval sprints.** During sprint intervals, the body trains above the lactate threshold (the exercise intensity at which lactic acid starts to accumulate in the bloodstream), and this increase in lactic acid stimulates HGH release. Researchers discovered that sprinting for 250 meters at 80% of maximal 100-meter speed elevated HGH, with no increase in levels of the catabolic stress hormone cortisol.

2. **Perform the long intervals first.** If you are performing intervals of various distances, it is best to do the longest, most difficult work at the beginning of your workout. Researchers looked at hormone response to both decreasing (400, 300, 200, 100 meters) and increasing (100, 200, 300, 400 meters) sprint interval protocols. The decreasing distance protocol had the greatest HGH response.

Strength Training

Strength training is a potent HGH stimulator and can be manipulated as follows in order to increase levels:

1. **Perform high-volume, short-rest workouts.** Instead of sitting around in between sets, try shortening your rest intervals for better results. Research shows that short rest periods and a large total volume of work are the two most important factors leading to a significant increase in HGH levels. Step out of your comfort zone and use heavier weights in the range of 75% to 85% of 1 rep maximum (1RM, which means the most you could lift for 1 single repetition). Keep rest intervals short between sets (less than one minute), and always use good form. If you are not sure how to perform an exercise or of the correct form, seek the instruction of a qualified personal trainer.

2. **Train like a bodybuilder.** Bodybuilders typically perform a greater number of sets per exercise than average (4 or more). Research shows that a protocol with 4 sets of 10 reps for each exercise induces a greater HGH release than is a workout using light weights or body weight, or a workout using very heavy weight but with fewer sets. The intensity should be kept at about 75% of 1RM for the best results. Keep rest intervals short to increase lactate (a salt derivative of lactic acid) and oxygen debt—two things that lead to an increase in growth hormone production and have a positive effect on both fat loss and muscle growth. Done correctly, the resistance-training workouts I provide in chapter 10 will stimulate HGH release.

3. **Emphasize the negative.** When training with weights, it is important to pay attention to the tempo of each rep. Lowering the weight too quickly will diminish the production of lactic acid important for HGH production. Periodically challenge yourself by lowering weights that are the equivalent of 100% of your 1RM for 4 to 6 reps. To do this safely, you must have a training partner spot you.

Nutrition and HGH

Nutrition also plays a role in HGH production, and the consumption of certain nutrients can impact HGH release. Complement your high-intensity training by consuming protein immediately after your workout. Sufficient intake of protein is essential for maximizing the muscle-building potential of exercise-related HGH release.

Sleep and HGH

HGH is affected not only by resistance training, cardio, and nutrition but by other external factors, such as sleep, as well.

Part of the repair and recovery process, sleep is imperative for the release of hormones such as HGH. You may have heard the expression "Burn fat while you sleep." You really can burn fat while you sleep, though only because of the lipolytic action of nocturnal HGH secretion and the subsequent fatty acid release made possible by it.

HGH secretion peaks late at night and is linked to sleep duration. Sleep deprivation reduces HGH secretion. Ensure you are getting the most from your sleep by following these simple tips:

1. **Sleep in complete darkness.** Even a small amount of light can disrupt the release of HGH.
2. **Maintain consistent sleep habits.** Go to bed and get up at the same time, even on the weekends. Avoid disrupting your body's natural sleep rhythms.
3. **Do not overeat before bed.** Excessive calories consumed pre-bedtime can make falling asleep uncomfortable and difficult for some people.
4. **Keep it quiet.** Keep the bedroom extremely quiet or use a white-noise generator.
5. **Keep it cool.** Keep a slightly cool temperature in the room, between 66°F and 72°F (19°C and 22°C).
6. **Practice stress-management techniques.** Meditate or pray before bed, and avoid watching television or a movie, or using your computer, or anything else that may increase stress and disrupt sleep.
7. **Avoid evening stimulants.** Eliminate stimulants like caffeine and nicotine, especially later in the day.
8. **Exercise.** Another reason to work out: exercise can help improve sleep.

What about HGH-Releasing Supplements?

A variety of nasal sprays, homeopathic formulas, sublinguals, and secretagogues are available without a prescription from supplement companies and health food stores. The problem is that they do not work. Forget these overhyped products and remember: there are no shortcuts. The strategies listed above are the best ways to maximize your body's natural production of HGH.

THYROID

When discussing hard-to-lose body fat, the subject of thyroid function invariably comes up. Most people know that an underactive thyroid (also known as hypothyroid) can often make losing body fat pretty difficult.

Low thyroid is not uncommon. Approximately 3% to 5% of the population may be affected by it at any given time—that's a pretty big number indeed. Hypothyroidism is much more common in women than in men.

So that you can better understand this problem, here's a quick overview of thyroid. There are two main thyroid hormones, T4 and T3. Your body releases these hormones via a small gland located near the front of your neck. The thyroid gland releases about twenty times more T4 than T3, but approximately one-third of this T4 gets converted into T3. Much more potent than T4, T3 has the biggest impact on metabolism.

High concentrations of T3 increase the number of beta receptors (those receptors that help us burn fat). You'll recall that the number of beta and alpha receptors in your body correlates to how easy (or difficult) it is to lose that fat, and we all tend to have fewer beta and more alpha receptors in our trouble spots, where it's hardest to shed the fat.

T3 also impacts your metabolic rate and how well your body burns fat from all areas. If you have low levels of T3, then despite your best efforts, you probably struggle with losing fat.

Are You Affected? Symptoms of Low Thyroid

Several symptoms may indicate hypothyroidism:

- Sudden, unexplained weight gain
- Difficulty losing weight despite proper nutrition and exercise
- Feelings of overall fatigue or weakness
- Depression
- Thinning hair and/or brittle nails
- Decreased libido
- Puffiness in hands, face, or feet
- Memory loss
- Muscle aches and pains
- Excessive tiredness
- Abnormal menstruation
- Slow heart rate
- Diminished taste and smell
- Intolerance to cold
- Bulging eyes

That's quite a list, and at any given time you (and I) are probably experiencing one or more of these symptoms! For example, I have a deep-rooted intolerance of cold weather and sometimes forget where I left my car keys, but I have no thyroid issues whatsoever. That's why it is always imperative that you rely on testing and avoid self-diagnosing using the Internet. Visit your doctor and ask to have your thyroid-stimulating hormone (TSH) levels tested. Like the name implies, TSH stimulates your thyroid and controls the release of both T3 and T4.

Elevated TSH typically suggests underactive thyroid. The normal spectrum for TSH is quite broad, ranging from 0.4 to 4.0 mlU/L. Again, have your levels tested by your doctor to ensure an accurate diagnosis.

Increasing Thyroid Naturally

If you want to be proactive, you can take some steps to ensure normal thyroid function:

1. **Consume iodine-rich foods.** Your body needs dietary iodine to properly synthesize thyroid hormones. An iodine deficiency will result in a lower production of T4. The recommended daily allowance for iodine is 150 micrograms per day for adult women and men. Augment your diet with iodine-rich foods, including iodized salt and sea salt (use in moderation), saltwater fish, seaweed, sesame seeds, seafood, kelp, dulse, and asparagus.

2. **Take regular diet breaks.** Excessive calorie restriction over an extended period (more than 14 consecutive days) can lead to diminished thyroid function because of reduced conversion of T4 to T3 in the liver. This is a bad thing, as T3 is the active form of thyroid that provides all the wonderful fat-burning benefits. If you are dieting, increasing your calories (including carbohydrates) once per week will prevent low thyroid.

Certain foods should be avoided if you have hypothyroidism:

- Processed and frozen ready-made foods
- White flour and white rice products (lacking in nutrients)
- All saturated fat and fried foods
- Soy protein in excessive amounts
- Hydrogenated oils, margarine, and shortening
- Fructose and high-fructose corn syrup (in excessive quantities, these can slow down thyroid function)
- Sugars, artificial sweeteners, and sweets (these can weaken the immune system)

Also avoid drinking and cooking with tap water, as the fluoride and chlorine found in it block iodine reception in the thyroid gland.

A number of chemicals can affect thyroid production as well. These include chemicals found in pesticides, herbicides, plastics, and even some skin creams and shampoos. Whenever possible, choose natural beauty products and thoroughly wash any fruit or vegetable you plan to eat that has the outer layer or skin intact.

Summing Things Up

Consuming iodine-rich food and taking regular diet breaks, along with avoiding the foods listed above, will help optimize your body's thyroid functioning, especially if you are working toward peak body composition. If you find that you have a true thyroid deficiency, the only likely remedy will come from proper medication via your doctor.

You now have a firm grasp on how your body burns fat and the hormones involved in the process. In the coming pages you will learn about the diet and training program that will remove your trouble spot fat. But first, I would like to dispel some of the most common myths about losing trouble spot fat.

5

Ditching the Diet Dogma

The weight-loss industry is fraught with enduring dogma and myths. Challenging these myths is always met with resistance, since most people prefer to remain comfortable with familiar and popular ideas than face the prospect that they were wrong and need to change. This is a shame—any one of the following myths could be holding you back from having the body you desire (or needlessly complicating your life). Let's take a look at some of the most common ones.

MYTH: A CALORIE IS A CALORIE

Many dieticians and trainers claim that when it comes to losing fat, it doesn't matter where your calories come from, just so long as you consume fewer than you burn. This is based on the incorrect notion that because a pound of fat is equal to 3500 calories of energy, all you need to do to lose a pound is to either (a) expend 3500 calories through activity or (b) reduce caloric intake by 3500 calories. According to this theory, you can eat nothing but candy bars and cookies and still lose weight, just so long as you comply with one of these deficit-inducing methods.

This archaic methodology is based on some seriously flawed science. First, it assumes that every morsel of food eaten is digested and its nutrients assimilated by the body—it isn't and they aren't. When the 19th-century chemist Wilbur Atwater devised the method for calculating the calorie content of food that's still used today, he used an *incinerator*. Incineration is vastly different from human digestion, and the efficiency of digestion varies widely between individuals.

Second, the quality of calories differs in terms of the body's hormonal response to various foods. The human body is not like a bomb calorimeter. The action of eating induces a hormonal response in the body. And protein, for instance, has a very different effect on hormones, satiation, and metabolism than do carbohydrates.

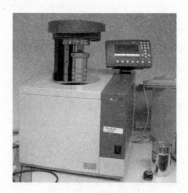

The bomb calorimeter

Is this what your digestive system looks like?
I didn't think so. But this is the machine used today
to "analyze" the calorie content of individual foods.

Third, food choices can induce negative responses in some individuals. For example, many people are allergic to wheat and dairy, and foods containing them can cause an inflammatory response and wreak hormonal havoc in them.

Calories do count when on a fat-loss program, but it is important to remember that the source of those calories matters as well.

MYTH: "FAT-BURNING ZONE" HEART RATE

The "fat-burning zone" is a prevailing myth within the fitness industry perpetuated by the manufacturers of cardio-training equipment, as evidenced by the "cardio zone" and "fat-burning zone" programs found on treadmills, bikes, and other machines.

This myth is actually based on a modicum of truth. Your body uses a mix of fat and carbohydrates to fuel the energy needs of your cells. When you exercise at a low intensity, your body preferentially uses fat for fuel. As the exercise intensity increases, so too does your body's dependence on muscle glycogen, until eventually the muscles are using only glycogen to fuel contraction.

Since more fat is used during low-intensity exercise, people often assume that it is best for burning fat, an idea that has given birth to the concept of the "fat-burning zone." However, while only a small amount of fat is used when exercising at a high intensity, just below the lactate threshold (when lactic acid starts to accumulate in the bloodstream), the rate of caloric expenditure and the *total number of calories expended* are much greater than they are when exercising at a lower intensity. High-intensity exercise better facilitates a calorie deficit and a greater overall amount of fat lost. It also induces a more profound release of the catecholamine hormones, which are necessary for mobilizing trouble spot fat.

So take the focus off working out in the low-intensity "fat-burning zone," and focus on increasing the effort expended during your workout.

MYTH: DO HIGH REPS FOR FAT-BURNING

High reps are for cutting, low reps are for bulking. This is a common belief held among most exercisers. It is also false.

One of the first things to understand is that you cannot "cut" or "define" a muscle with strength training. Performing endless repetitions will not add "detail," nor "shape" or "sculpt" your muscles.

The purpose of weight training while on a fat-loss program is muscle preservation, not calorie expenditure. Don't get me wrong, strength training and increased energy expenditure will contribute somewhat to your fat-loss effort. But you shouldn't design lifting programs aimed solely at burning fat. Performing high-rep exercise with light weights will do nothing to help preserve muscle mass while you're on a diet and might even lead to muscle wasting if the volume is excessive. If you do perform this type of training as a form of high-intensity interval training (HIIT), be sure to include days of heavy-weight, low-volume work in order to avoid muscle loss, and use diet to induce the calorie deficit.

MYTH: EAT SIX SMALL MEALS PER DAY

We have all heard this dictum, and many of us are still living by it: "Eating small, frequent meals throughout the day increases metabolism." This is, in fact, false. There is no evidence to support the idea that skipping a single meal or even a day's worth of meals does anything to metabolic rate. Your body's metabolism simply doesn't operate that quickly, and recent research into fasting even shows a slight (approximately 5%) increase in metabolic rate during the initial period of fasting! Other studies suggest that compared with eating six times per day, eating three high-protein meals per day is better for maintaining levels of satiety.

The concept of increased meal frequency and enhanced metabolism was born from the concept of the thermic effect of food (TEF). Whenever you eat, your metabolism is boosted above its baseline while your body expends energy to digest what you consumed, convert it to energy, and dispose of it. Approximately 30% of the protein calories you consume are burned via TEF, 15% to 20% of carbohydrate calories, and 3% to 5% of fat calories.

What's important to note is that the rate of TEF—the amount of energy required to process and digest the food we eat—is dependent on total calories eaten, not on meal frequency. If you eat five 400-calorie meals, the TEF would be identical to eating two 1000-calorie meals, provided the ratio of proteins, carbs, and fats was the same. The idea that skipping breakfast or a single snack or meal slows metabolism or induces a starvation response is simply not true. In my own experience, and based on my observations working with clients, success is possible by eating one, two, or three—and even all the way up to seven!— times per day. Any meal is negotiable, the only exception being post-workout nutrition—that is not negotiable.

I do believe that eating more frequently is beneficial for those who have higher caloric requirements and when calories are increased during a muscle-building phase. For example, athletes may need 6000 calories (or more) per day to fuel their training, and for them, eating five 1200-calorie meals may work better than eating two 3000-calorie meals. Because of insulin's anabolic properties, the frequent insulin spikes that come from eating multiple times per day may be beneficial for those individuals seeking an increase in muscle mass. Just keep in mind that the most important component to any successful nutrition plan is adherence. The plan that will work is the one that you can follow.

This doesn't mean that eating small, frequent meals is bad. In fact, I do it almost every day, and many of my most successful clients do as well. What this does mean is that you don't have to obsess over when your next meal is coming. A better approach is to focus on hitting your calorie and protein requirements for the day and spreading your meals out in such a way that you are able to stick to your healthy diet and not fall off the wagon every other day.

MYTH: EATING BEFORE BED MAKES YOU FAT

Just like skipping breakfast is wrongly associated with higher body fat percentage, late-night eating is associated by many people with increased body fat. This too is a myth. Since calories are equal, meal timing has no impact on body weight.

A recent study compared two meal patterns, one group eating most of the daily calories earlier in the day, and the other group eating most of the calories later in the day. Researchers discovered that those who ate more calories in the morning lost more weight; however, the extra weight was in the form of muscle mass. The subjects who ate in the late evening had less muscle loss, and this resulted in a greater decrease in body fat percentage. Some experts preach the benefits of fasting past six o'clock in the evening, claiming that doing so will speed up weight loss. The only reason this method sometimes works is that it eliminates evening snacking and forces a person to eat less total calories for the day.

The truth is, the time of day that you eat your meals won't affect your body composition.

MYTH: HIGH-PROTEIN DIETS ARE BAD FOR YOUR KIDNEYS

A common criticism of high-protein diets is that they are damaging to the kidneys. For healthy people, this statement is unfounded; it applies only to those with preexisting kidney damage. Although eating large amounts of protein does increase the workload imposed on the kidneys, it does not naturally follow that the kidneys will be damaged.

The main concern with increased protein consumption is the potential for metabolic acidosis, a condition that occurs when you eat too many acid-producing foods and the body creates too much acid in response. Because most protein sources are acid-forming, the acid load needs to be counteracted by alkalizing foods. You can accomplish this by eating lots of fruits and vegetables, especially dark green vegetables like spinach, kale, and broccoli, as well as alkaline fruits such as cherries, grapes, and kiwis.

Other dietary strategies that can help shift you to an alkaline state include:

- Eliminating processed grains and minimizing intake of whole-grain breads and cereals.
- Limiting dairy intake to fermented selections from grass-fed animals.
- Eliminating cheese.
- Squeezing fresh lemon and lime juice into your drinking water.
- Supplementing your diet with a green food supplement such as greens+ and glutamine.
- Taking 5000 IUs (international units) of vitamin D and 500 milligrams of magnesium daily to enhance calcium absorption and bone formation, both of which are negatively impacted by a high-acid-load diet.

MYTH: ALCOHOL MAKES YOU FAT

The concept that alcohol can make you fat contains a modicum of truth. When you drink alcohol, it is converted into acetate by the liver. This conversion takes priority over metabolizing other nutrients, and this can inhibit lipolysis and enable dietary fats to be stored with ease. Yet, despite inhibiting fat burning, alcohol *alone* cannot cause fat gain, as there is no metabolic pathway that can make fat out of alcohol with any efficiency. It's all the junk food people eat in conjunction with drinking that causes fat gain.

The hype over moderate alcohol consumption and health is unfounded. To begin with, alcohol is not as calorie-dense as once believed. Although it starts out at a rather high 7 calories per gram, it takes a lot of energy to process and actually nets out closer to 5 (which is just slightly more than protein). Next, when one looks at the research, it can almost be said that moderate alcohol consumption is healthier than no alcohol at all. Some benefits include improvements in insulin sensitivity, reduction in rates of cancer, and even longer life! Things can deteriorate, though, since a high volume of alcohol can lower testosterone, but you really have to drink a lot for this to occur.

The negative effects of moderate alcohol consumption have been exaggerated by the fitness community. That being said, there are some points to keep in mind when deciding on what to drink.

How to Drink Alcohol *and* Lose Fat

Here are some tips to keep in mind when consuming alcohol:

- **Limit carbohydrate-rich alcohol sources.** These include beer and drinks made with fruit juice.
- **Stick to the darker beers** if you're a beer lover, like I am. They are not as easy to slam back, and they're full of beneficial antioxidants. The downside to beer is that

it increases estrogen levels and for this reason should be consumed only on occasion.

- **Choose dry wines.** These are very low in carbs, as opposed to sweet wines.
- **Choose low-carb spirits.** These include cognac, tequila, rum, scotch, gin, vodka, and whiskey—all are good choices.
- **Don't mix alcohol with regular soda.** Use diet soda or soda water instead. Avoid tonic water; it is surprisingly high in sugar.
- **Keep starch-based carbs very low.** Avoid breads, pasta, rice, and so on; instead, stick to eating vegetables and protein.
- **Don't eat fruit with your alcohol.** When your liver is busy processing the alcohol, fructose can remain in circulation, leaving it free to react with proteins or fats to form AGEs (advanced glycation end-products) that increase inflammation in the body.
- **Dramatically reduce your intake of fats.** Never consume fatty foods and alcohol together. Alcohol reduces your body's ability to oxidize fatty acids, preventing it from using fat for fuel. To avoid fat storage, don't consume greasy foods with your favorite drink.
- **Eat as much protein as you want.** Just make sure to get your protein from lean sources, such as low-fat cottage cheese, protein powder, chicken, turkey, tuna, or egg whites.
- **Don't replace your post-workout protein shake with a beer.** In fact, consuming any alcohol immediately post-exercise will negatively affect your recovery.

I am not suggesting that it is fine to drink until you drop like a freshman at college. In fact, no strategy can negate the effects of an all-out booze bender. Studies show that when excessive amounts of alcohol are consumed (three drinks or more), there is an increase in cortisol and estrogen, and a decrease in next-day performance. Consuming one to two drinks did not appear to produce any ill effects. All this being said, it is a fact of life that some people are going to drink too much from time to time, and when this happens, some simple strategies can reverse the damage:

1. **Drink green tea on days that you drink, as well as the day after.** Green tea contains catechins, which inhibit the absorption of alcohol while reducing inflammation.
2. **Supplement with curcumin.** Curcumin (found in turmeric) is excellent for reducing inflammation and helps protect the liver from alcohol-related damage.
3. **Use milk thistle.** Milk thistle helps speed the elimination of toxins and is highly regarded for its liver-protecting properties.

If you follow these rules, you can drink freely once (or twice) per week with no fear of fat gain. To be clear, I am not advocating excess alcohol consumption. But I myself enjoy an occasional drink or two. When consumed responsibly, alcohol poses no threat to your health or waistline.

MYTH: SKIPPING MEALS CAUSES MUSCLE LOSS

This myth is based on the irrational fear that if you happen to skip a meal, your body will break down muscle tissue for use as an energy source. This is not something anybody has to worry about. Protein is absorbed at a very slow rate, and after a large, high-protein meal, amino acids trickle into your bloodstream over the course of several hours. This effect can be quite profound, especially when you eat slow-digesting proteins or a combination of protein, fat, and carbohydrates. In this case, a single high-protein meal may release amino acids for more than 16 hours, thus negating any chance of muscle loss.

Some studies even show *improvements* to body composition when meals are consumed sporadically, as opposed to every 2 to 3 hours, as once believed. This does not mean you should adopt an "eat what you want, when you want" approach to your meal patterns. If you do go more than 24 hours without food, stored liver glycogen will become depleted and catabolism (muscle tissue breakdown) will become an issue, as *de novo gluconeogenesis* will occur. This is when amino acids from muscle tissue are converted into glucose for use as energy by the body. The best way to prevent de novo gluconeogenesis is to never go more than 24 hours without eating protein and to eat sufficient amounts of protein with every meal.

MYTH: SATURATED FAT IS BAD FOR YOU

One of my favorite television programs is *Conspiracy Theory*, with former Minnesota governor and WWF wrestling star Jesse Ventura. No matter what you believe to be true about 9/11, the Kennedy assassination, or Roswell, New Mexico, Jesse will have you taking a moment to say "Hmmm . . ."

I admit to sometimes being a conspiracy theorist myself, especially when it comes to some of the recommendations made by our mainstream medical community. It is hard to deny that there is a fatal flaw in a system where drug companies can influence the decisions of doctors who write the prescriptions. A good example of this is all the propaganda surrounding cholesterol levels, saturated fat intake, and heart disease. For years, the message being preached has been to avoid eggs, butter, bacon, and other foods high in saturated fat or you will pay the price with heart disease and high cholesterol. As a result, millions of people have abandoned these foods for high-carb substitutions in the form of refined-grain products, together with a dose of statin drugs to keep their cholesterol levels in check.

Turns out that "they" were wrong. In an article published in the *American Journal of Clinical Nutrition* in 2010, researchers looked at 21 prospective epidemiological studies with a total of more than 347,000 test subjects. Their conclusions: absolutely no association between saturated fat and heart disease.

The truth is that consuming saturated fat does not increase the risk of heart disease. Although eating saturated fat does raise cholesterol, it elevates levels of the "good" HDL form. In terms of LDL or "bad" cholesterol levels, consuming saturated fat changes the LDL from small, dense LDL (very bad) to large LDL, which is benign.

This fact should remove any unfounded fear you may have about my recommendation to eat healthy fats in the form of coconut oil, organic butter, cheese, or—my personal favorite—whole eggs, among others. All these foods are high in nutrients. The bottom line is this: saturated fat does not cause heart disease, and foods that are naturally high in saturated fat are good for you (unless you have hypothyroidism).

MYTH: YOU CAN DIGEST ONLY 30 GRAMS OF PROTEIN PER MEAL

A long-standing tenet held by those in the fitness industry is that the body can use only 30 grams of protein per meal, and the excess is either oxidized or excreted. This guideline has led many trainees to painstakingly measure the amount of protein eaten in each meal and even endure the hassle of consuming multiple doses of protein throughout the day, in the belief that this will maximize muscle growth and retention.

This concept dovetails nicely with the other long-standing myth that you have to eat at least six times per day in order to keep the body's metabolism revving high. Such dogma has, of course, been proven false. There is no known rate limit for protein digestion. In fact, recent research has shown the upper limit of protein digestibility to be much higher than 30 grams per meal and more in line with the *total* daily protein requirements.

In other words, if your daily requirement of protein is 150 grams, then that amount could be digested, absorbed, and utilized by eating it all in one meal, thus negating the need for small, multiple servings throughout the day.

Fundamentally, protein utilization can differ according to a person's muscle mass and activity level. The more muscle you have and the more often you exercise, the greater your need for dietary protein. I typically set individual protein requirements at 0.75 to 1 gram per pound of body weight daily.

In terms of application, I believe it's effective to consume protein before *and* after resistance-training workouts. A good rule of thumb is to aim for consuming approximately one-quarter of your body weight in grams in both the pre- and post-exercise meals. On non-exercise or cardio-only days, combine or split up your total protein allotment according to your meal-frequency preference and your body's ability to comfortably digest high-protein meals. This will provide you with some freedom and flexibility when planning your daily meals.

MYTH: LOW-CARB DIETS ARE BAD

One of the worst recommendations you can give a person who is trying to lose body fat is to increase the intake of high-carb foods and grains in any form. The agricultural revolution is a relatively recent event in human evolution, and our genes have yet to adapt to the change in dietary habits from those of our hunter-gatherer ancestors. Grains, and in particular wheat, can cause numerous problems, not the least of which are gluten sensitivity and issues with nutrient absorption. Grain products also increase insulin levels, which, as you have recently learned, is detrimental to mobilizing trouble spot fat deposits. When used strategically, low-carb diets can achieve many successful outcomes, including:

- Reducing body fat at an accelerated rate.
- Increasing HDL (good) cholesterol levels while inducing the transformation of LDL cholesterol from the harmful small, dense form to the large form, which is benign.
- Lowering blood pressure significantly.
- Lowering blood sugar and improving symptoms of diabetes.
- Increasing compliance to diet because of greater appetite control.

This is not to say that carbohydrate foods are inherently bad. Quite the contrary, in fact. Consuming high-carb meals strategically can help you avoid most of the negative adaptations that can come from following a low-carb diet over the long term. Unfortunately, most of the recommendations regarding "healthy" carbohydrate consumption and low-fat intake are causing more harm than good.

MYTH: MEN AND WOMEN RESPOND TO DIET AND EXERCISE EXACTLY THE SAME WAY

Ask any experienced trainer and he or she will tell you that women have a more difficult time losing body fat than men do. For all the years I have been helping people improve their body composition, I cannot recall a single instance when a man had a difficult time making significant improvements. This is not to say that men find it easier implementing the necessary lifestyle changes required for optimal results. Instead, it appears that a man's body simply reacts differently to those changes than a woman's.

It is pretty obvious that when it comes to body composition, there are some significant differences between the sexes. For starters, women generally have a higher percentage of body fat than men. Also, women store more fat in the hip and thigh regions, whereas men store more fat in the visceral depot of the abdomen. And this is just what can be seen at a glance. Of course, digging a little deeper we can see that, when dieting, there are many more differences between the sexes. Here are a few to consider.

When Dieting, Women's Bodies Reduce Thermogenesis at a Faster Rate Than Men's

In a study published by the American Physiological Society, researchers concluded that during periods of calorie restriction, females deactivate thermogenesis (body heat generated by stimulating the metabolism and burning calories) to a greater degree than do males. Researchers hypothesize that this ability exists as a means to improve the odds of survival of the species when food is limited. When a woman goes on a diet, her metabolism may slow at a faster rate than a man's under the same conditions.

After Eating, Men Store More Visceral Fat and Women Store More Subcutaneous Fat

It turns out that women preferentially shuttle fat toward subcutaneous deposits—the fat that is very visible just beneath the skin. On the other hand, men tend to shuttle fat more readily to visceral deposits—the more dangerous fat that surrounds organs.

Women Store More Nutrients in Lower-Body Fat Than Men Do

After a meal, blood flow and transport of fats to the lower body are greater in women than in men. The old saying "A moment on the lips, a lifetime on the hips" may be true after all.

In the Post-Exercise Period, Men Mobilize Fat More Efficiently Than Women Do

A recent study examining the way men and women break down fat into free fatty acids in the post-exercise period shows that, after exercise, fat mobilization and metabolism are enhanced to a greater extent in men than in women.

Don't worry; I do have some good news if you are a woman . . .

During Exercise, Women Burn More Fat for Fuel, Men Burn More Carbohydrates

In a study published in the *Journal of Applied Physiology*, researchers looked at fuel metabolism in men and women during and after long-duration exercise. They discovered that women burn more fat when exercising at lower intensities than men do and may be more sensitive to the fat-burning action of the catecholamines, which are released during a good workout.

As you can see, the cards are stacked unfairly, and women do have more of a challenge when it comes to losing body fat. This also means that there are very few excuses for us guys, and we need to be supportive of our better halves. Women should not give up, of course. All this means is that you have to eat and train smarter than a man, and in the coming chapters I show you exactly how to do just that.

MYTH: "I HAVE A SLOW METABOLISM"

I hear this one all the time, and most folks have accepted it as a legitimate reason for gaining excess weight. Your metabolism is the process your body uses to obtain energy from the foods and beverages you consume. Chemical reactions in your body break down these substances into sugars and fatty acids for you to use as energy or to store in various tissues. In some people, a condition known as metabolic syndrome can develop, resulting in an increase in abdominal fat, in blood glucose levels, and in high blood pressure while fasting. The good news is that this condition can be prevented and even reversed with the right lifestyle modifications.

Otherwise healthy people who complain of having a "slow metabolism" don't have a metabolism problem. They have an activity problem. It is common to hear people claim that their metabolism slowed down when they got older. This may be true, but usually it's because they themselves slowed down. Some 60% of your metabolism is "fixed," the other 40% variable.

You have control over four variables that will serve to increase your metabolism.

Resting Metabolic Rate (RMR)

Your resting metabolic rate (RMR) is the energy your body needs to sustain its most basic functions and is determined largely by your lean body mass (LBM). Most folks assume "lean body mass" refers to how much muscle one carries, but that is only partly correct. Lean body mass is everything in your body that is not fat. This includes organs, blood, bones, skin, and, of course, muscle. Although muscle mass accounts for about 40% of RMR, the other 60% is a factor of brain and organ function. Because we can't increase the size of our brains or organs, it makes sense to train with resistance in order to increase LBM, as this will increase your RMR. Men typically have a higher RMR than women largely because of differences in LBM.

Thermic Effect of Food

As we know, a certain amount of energy is required to process and digest the foods we eat. This is known as the thermic effect of food, or TEF. Protein has the highest TEF at about 30%, followed by carbohydrates, and then fats. Because of its high thermic effect and the fact that protein is very satiating, increasing protein intake should be one of the first changes you make to your diet. Alcohol is also quite thermic (similar to protein), and this is one of the reasons it isn't as detrimental to your diet results as you may have been led to believe (let the celebrations begin).

Activity Level

This tends to be the variable that meets with the greatest amount of resistance. What a shame that is, since increased activity results in increased calories burned during the activity and afterward (through a process called excess post-exercise oxygen consumption, or EPOC). The number of calories burned during activity is largely dependent on the amount of work performed, so don't make the mistake of thinking that you burned 500 calories by walking around the block. The truth is, it takes a lot of effort to burn a significant number of calories, and most estimations you see on treadmills and other machines at the gym are horribly inaccurate. Metabolic resistance training, an example of which you will find in chapter 8's Protocol 3, produces the highest rate of EPOC, which is a major reason it is so effective for fat loss when done correctly.

Thermogenesis

Increased thermogenesis, or heat production, in the body can be accomplished relatively painlessly and can have a significant impact on metabolism. For example, the simple act of fidgeting can raise your body temperature and so burn several hundred extra calories per day. This is also known as non-exercise activity thermogenesis, or NEAT.

Generally, the more you exercise, the more food you should be eating, and the faster your metabolism will be. The opposite of this also holds true. If you want to slow your metabolism, eat like a squirrel and sit on the couch all day watching reruns. There is one important caveat. Not everybody's metabolism reacts to calorie intake the same way. Some genetically advantaged people increase metabolic rate faster during periods of increased calorie intake, and these same blessed folks have metabolisms that take longer to slow when calories are decreased. We probably all know someone who seems to get away with murder at the dining room table and still looks great. Someone like that simply has a brain that reacts more favorably to changes in calorie intake.

Kind of reminds me of a good-looking trust-fund baby or the person who just won the $300-million Powerball lottery—they got lucky. The rest of us simply have to suck it up, do it the old-fashioned way, and earn our results. And that's fine by me.

6

Body Recomposition
What Matters Most

My friend Shaun is an expert copywriter—one of those people who writes promotional material for a product or service idea, say, with the aim of persuading the reader or viewer to make a purchase. If you have ever found yourself compelled to buy something after reading an article or watching a commercial, you have experienced firsthand the power of good copywriting. It can literally mean the difference between $100 in sales and $100,000. It's that powerful. Last year, I hired Shaun to write a sales letter for me, and in the process of its creation I was introduced to the art of copywriting and the power of the written word. It turns out that when it comes to the weight-loss market, some words work better than others at persuading consumers to open their wallets. These include:

Trim
Tighten
Firm
Tone
Shape
Slim

Now, here is my issue with these words—they are all meaningless! There is no quantifiable method of assessment to accurately measure muscle "tone" or "shape." Your goal should not be to trim, tighten, tone, firm, or shape. This is all BS marketing talk designed to sell you some useless contraption on late-night TV. Instead, your goal is body *recomposition*. This could mean:

The loss of 20 pounds of fat.
The gain of 10 pounds of muscle.
The loss of 5% body fat.
The loss of 4 inches of fat from your waist.
The goal to fit into the pants you wore in high school.

There is nothing abstract about these goals. They are quantifiable and can be tracked until completion. In the science community there is a popular axiom: "Everything that is measured gets managed." The trick is to know what to measure. Most weight-loss programs fail before they begin by focusing solely on weight loss. In this chapter, I teach you how to pay attention to the important stuff while ignoring the distractions that can take you off track.

TELL ME, WHAT DO YOU *REALLY* WANT?

Do you want more muscle, less fat, or both? Regardless of what the answer is, chances are you are not measuring your progress the right way. Do not focus on pounds gained or lost. Focus on building muscle and losing fat—in other words, body *recomposition*. Doing the least to get the most—this is the goal. Too much dieting results in a negative hormonal feedback; too much exercise leads to injury. You want to do the least amount of each that will produce the best possible results. To accomplish this, you need to know what to measure and track.

Women are notorious for obsessing over the numbers they see when they step on a scale. The typical man could tell you who won the big game last night but would be hard-pressed to tell you what he weighs. Yet, I have met scores of women who weigh themselves not once but multiple times per day. It's almost as if the act of weighing one's self were going to speed up the whole process. As you are about to discover, thinking this way is a big mistake.

BODY RECOMPOSITION

Your body consists of many elements that make up total body weight, including water, muscle, blood, bone, tissue, organs, undigested food, and . . . ahem . . . poop. Cleansing diets and products focus on your losing the latter (mainly poop), whereas the most aggressive, extreme low-calorie diets end up causing you to lose more of the former (water and muscle). Losing undigested food matter and poop is a good thing but can hardly be called a success in terms of fat loss. Losing significant amounts of muscle is a complete disaster and should be avoided at all costs. What you are looking for is the loss of body fat with a minimal loss of muscle tissue. Don't kid yourself— when trying to rid your body of trouble spot fat, there will likely be some collateral damage in the form of muscle loss. After all, losing fat requires a calorie deficit, and this puts the body in a catabolic state. This is why so many athletes turn to anabolic steroids. These steroids are incredible at preventing muscle breakdown and make dieting a total breeze. When you are on anabolic steroids, you can severely reduce calories while exercising intensely and lose tons of fat without muscle loss. This isn't the case when you are a natural-training athlete like you and me. If we were to diet and work out like crazy, we would quickly overtrain and lose significant amounts of lean mass. I am going to teach you how to minimize these losses and possibly even turn the tables by slightly increasing lean muscle mass while simultaneously slashing your body fat percentage. My goal is for you to keep muscle loss to a bare minimum while maximizing the release of fat from your trouble spots.

You see, body recomposition (the term I use for simultaneous fat loss and muscle gain) is not impossible; it's just tricky. Most conventional methods don't work because they approach the goal primarily through training, which isn't the best way. This is evidenced by the multitude of infomercials that flood the networks each January. All the training in the world won't do squat at removing trouble spot fat. You must adjust your diet too.

To achieve body recomposition, we are going to do both.

EVERYTHING THAT IS MEASURED GETS MANAGED

In my experience, a typical conversation during a fitness assessment goes like this:

"How many calories are you eating each day?" I ask.

"Not many. I hardly eat, and when I do, it's all healthy stuff," Newbie answers.

"What's your percent body fat?"

"I have no idea . . ." Newbie says.

"What does your exercise program look like?"

"I do treadmill and yoga and light weights three times per week."

"What exercises do you do, and for how many sets and reps?"

"I don't know. I just work out really hard . . ."

This approach doesn't work, and the reason is simple. Nothing gets measured, so nothing gets managed. Legions of people approach exercise this way, and the interesting thing is that most people deal with their relationships, finances, and life this way too! The reason the laissez-faire approach is so popular is simple: it works—but only at the beginning.

When you first embark on an exercise or diet program, everything seems to work. You lose a few pounds. You gain a bit of muscle strength and definition. You feel great and think that you have this whole losing fat thing all figured out.

And then it stops working. Suddenly your progress stops just as quickly as it started, and you have no idea how to fix it. It's like trying to save money without any figure in mind, and without access to your bank statements. Without measurable steps and a clearly defined goal, you are merely shooting wildly into the dark, hoping you will hit your mark. This is not the way to achieve any goal, let alone that of losing the trouble spot fat that has plagued you for years. Here is the better approach.

STEP 1: KNOW YOUR DESTINATION

Why did you buy this book? Given its title, *Trouble Spot Fat Loss*, I can only assume it is because you have some fat that you are having a tough time getting rid of. But if your goal is simply "to lose some fat," you are going to have to be a lot more concise than that. To be achievable, the outcome must be clearly defined and measurable—your goal needs to be quantifiable. Adding words such as "toning" or "firming" isn't enough. Your goal of body recomposition can be measured only by calculating your body fat percentage. The following figures will help you decide where you want to be, and where you need to start in terms of the programs offered in this book.

Level 5

Male: 21% to 30%+ body fat
Female: 26% to 40%+ body fat

Men at this level have no separation of muscles and no vascularity (visible veins). The waist is substantially larger than the hips. There is fat covering all areas of the body (though it is not uncommon for men with a high body fat percentage to have very lean calf muscles). Women at the high end of this range display significant fat storage in all areas of the body but especially around the hips, thighs, stomach, and arms. For both sexes, the high end of this range is considered to be an unhealthy level of body fat and can make performing everyday activities difficult.

Level 4

Male: 15% to 20% body fat
Female: 21% to 25% body fat

These levels are average. A typical man in this category displays limited definition in his muscles but still has some shape to them. A woman at this level will have some curves without being considered overweight. Both sexes in this range will have significant fat deposits, with a small amount of visible separation between the major muscle groups. At this level you are still working to lower body fat percentage in order to get to trouble spot fat areas.

Level 3

Male: 10% to 14% body fat
Female: 16% to 20% body fat

Things are looking very good here. Some muscle definition and vascularity is evident, particularly in men, and when the lighting is good, you will even see visible definition in the abdominal area. This is considered a very low body fat percentage for women, and they will display muscle definition in the legs, arms, and shoulders. Most men look excellent at this level and would be considered to have the quintessential "beach body." Possible trouble spot fat areas that remain at this level include the abdomen and love handles in men, and the abdomen, thighs, and buttocks in women. Men and women at this level look very healthy and fit.

Level 2
Male: 6% to 9% body fat
Female: 12% to 15% body fat
This is the level that is just a touch less extreme than what you'd see in a competition bodybuilder. Muscle definition is prominent, and faces will appear to be somewhat gaunt because of a reduction in facial fat. Men will have veins appearing in the arms and possibly the lower abs. Women will have noticeable separation between muscles in legs and arms as well. This is an excellent look for both men and women who want to do a photo shoot with minimal clothing. Possible trouble spot fat areas that remain at this level include lower abdominal area in men, and thighs and buttocks in women.

Level 1
Male: 3% to 5% body fat
Female: 9% to 11% body fat
At this level, you are at or very close to competition body-builder shape. Veins are visible in the lower abs, and there is very little (if any) subcutaneous fat left. At this level, a man will have such low body fat that even his glutes would have striations, whereas a woman will display vascularity, striations, and separation in her muscles. Women who achieve such low body fat are also unable to menstruate. Both men and women at this level tend to not have any trouble spot fat left. This is not a

healthy level of body fat and should be sustained for a very brief period only, if it's reached at all.

STEP 2: CHOOSE YOUR TOOLS

I have an embarrassing confession to share with you. I don't know how much I weigh. I have a ballpark idea, of course, but I rarely step on a scale. But I can tell you that my current body fat percentage is 10 and my waist is 32 inches. I track these numbers using very simple tools, and I suggest you do the same. When a person is obese, the goal is simply to drop weight, and a scale will suffice as the measurement tool. But we are concerned with body recomposition, which is the dropping of fat pounds while maintaining or increasing lean body mass. For these purposes, a scale is a rather blunt measurement device and provides incomplete information. So instead, let's focus on two forms of measurement: percent body fat and girth measurements.

Calculating Your Percent Body Fat

There are three methods you can use to measure your percent body fat:

1. **Online tools that calculate percent body fat based on body measurements, height, and weight.** There are several online tools that can help you measure your body fat percentage . Look for one that doesn't rely solely on height and weight but also includes measurements because I want you to get used to assessing your body composition based on size and muscle mass more than weight. You will find a free such tool at http://www.ebodi.com/MyNutrition/WellnessAnalysis.aspx.

   When measuring your weight, remove your clothing first. Date and record your measurements in a diary or logbook so that you can watch the numbers decrease over time, which is ultimately what matters most.

2. **Skin-fold calipers.** When done correctly, this is the preferred method for most personal trainers. Most body fat is stored subcutaneously, beneath the skin. By using skin-fold calipers to pinch folds of skin and fat at precise areas of the body, a skilled tester can determine with great accuracy the body fat percentage of a man or woman. Be sure to have the same person test you each time, as results will vary depending on the technique used. For an online skin-fold calculator, visit http://www.exrx.net/Calculators/BodyComp.html. If you browse around, you will find more information on this site about testing procedures too.

3. **Infrared (Futrex).** The Futrex device sends a beam of infrared light into your biceps muscle. Fluctuations in the wavelength of the beam are used to estimate body fat percentage. One of the great things about this method is the ease of use—it's a breeze! The popularity of this method is increasing, and many health professionals now have them in their offices. Ask your doctor, chiropractor, or other health-care professional to test you.

A Note on the Body Mass Index

The body mass index (BMI) is a measure of body fat based on height and weight. The problem with the BMI is that it does not take into account fat versus lean tissue. The BMI incorrectly diagnoses about 25% of the population and is completely useless for athletes. For example, an athlete who is 6 feet tall and weighs 205 pounds will have a BMI of 27.8, indicating that he is overweight. Yet he may have 8% body fat and be in great shape. Forget about the BMI and focus on body fat percentage instead.

———

I also suggest that in addition to monitoring your body fat percentage, you do the following:

1. **Take a "before" picture of yourself.** Then take another picture (using similar lighting and clothing) every 30 days. Pictures will often show progress that you just do not notice by looking in the mirror every day.
2. **Take measurements.** Measurements are an excellent indicator of progress. Get a tailor's tape and measure and record the following every four to six weeks:

   Neck
   Shoulder
   Chest
   Upper arms
   Waist
   Hips
   Thigh
   Calf

   And use a scale to measure body weight.

Points to Consider

Regardless of the method of measurement you choose, keep these important points in mind:

1. **Control the variables and maintain consistency of measurement.** Choose your preferred method of measurement and never deviate from it. A body fat test performed using skin-fold calipers will likely yield a result different from that of a test performed using a Futrex device. Maintain consistency in your method of measurement and have the same person perform

the skin fold test on you each time, if possible. In addition, record the time of day the test is performed and try to have it done at the same time throughout the process.

2. **Consider hydration and your monthly cycle.** Hydration levels can create significant discrepancies in your measurements. For this reason I prefer to test first thing in the morning after voiding the bladder and bowels. Women need to be mindful of where they are in their menstrual cycle, as this can impact water retention as well. Certain medications, including NSAIDs, corticosteroids, birth control pills, and blood pressure drugs, are notorious for increasing water retention, as is flying in an aircraft.

3. **Remove your piercings.** According to Chinese and ayurvedic medicine, body piercings can impact your endocrine system and have a negative effect on site-specific body fat deposits. Although acupuncture can provide support in the treatment of obesity, a wrongly placed piercing can have the opposite result. Navel piercings in particular should be avoided, especially if you are trying to lose trouble spot fat from your midsection. The insertion of foreign objects into the central meridian of the body will increase cortisol production and localized fat deposits.

PART THREE
YOUR BODY
MINUS THE FAT

7

Carb Fasting

The Fastest Way to Lose 10 Pounds of Fat

I like to stay up-to-date on everything that's new and happening in the world of health and fitness, and this means that I attend a lot of industry trade shows. These shows often feature various "celebrity" speakers, many of whom are personal trainers or dieticians. Having spent some time in the world of "celebrity" training myself, I can honestly say I despise the term "celebrity" being used to label anything. To me it seems that if you feel the need to tell people you are a celebrity, then you are *not* a celebrity. Anyway, one of these folks was on stage telling people that diets don't work. This person (who will remain anonymous) went on to say that with his approach, there was no need to monitor food intake, and all that was required was a simple cleansing product and the ability to eat intuitively. I remember thinking that this person was clearly delusional and had never taken the theory into the field of practical application.

Eating intuitively sounds like a good idea and even makes sense. After all, everybody knows by now that eating cake and donuts and washing them down with soda pop is a one-way ticket to fat city. But if everyone is intuitively aware of this, why aren't the companies that produce such products out of business?

The answer is simple. People like consuming this stuff, and if you tell them they can't have it, they want it even more. Trying to get people to eat like a caveman 24/7 looks good on paper but fails miserably in the real world. Of course, some individuals enjoy eating like squirrels their whole lives, but I have discovered that not only is this type of monklike sacrifice generally unrealistic, it's also unnecessary and can actually impede fat-loss progress.

Back in chapter 3, I explained the process by which your body releases and burns stored fatty acids. You may recall that three conditions must be met in order for your body to lose trouble spot fat:

1. You must be in a calorie deficit on most (but not all) days.
2. You must reduce carbohydrate intake (and lower insulin) in order to inhibit your alpha receptors.
3. You must exercise with sufficient intensity and duration to increase catecholamine output, beta receptor stimulation, and subsequent release and burning of fatty acids.

In this chapter we'll deal with the second of these conditions—reducing carbohydrate intake. Hold on, I know what you're thinking and, no, I'm not suggesting you follow a low-carb diet, like those popular in the 1980s. With this method, eating your favorite carbohydrate foods is not an option—it's a necessity!

CARBOHYDRATE FASTING: THE EASIEST, FASTEST, MOST PAIN-FREE WAY TO REDUCE CARBOHYDRATES

You will not lose your trouble spot fat eating a high-carbohydrate diet. Even if you are in a calorie deficit, the insulin response to eating a carbohydrate-based diet will inhibit the release of your hardest-to-lose trouble spot fat. I can hear the calorie-balance people crying, "All that matter is calories in minus calories out," and I acknowledge that there's some validity to this, but, as we've talked about, they are only partly correct. For an obese person just starting out, calorie balance *is* all that matters. But once you rid yourself of your *easy-to-lose* fat and are left with fat that just won't budge (trouble spot fat), you need to change your approach and consider the hormonal response that occurs whenever you eat.

Recall my saying that the human body is not a bomb calorimeter. There is more to the equation than simply calories in minus calories out. As with all things, the physics law of "Every action has an equal and opposite reaction" applies. The action of eating foods induces the reaction of hormonal response in the body. The hormonal response to protein, carbohydrates, and fat are each vastly different, especially when it comes to satiety and the catecholamines' effect on alpha and beta receptors.

Dietary carbohydrates must be lowered substantially in order to naturally inhibit your alpha receptors; the duration of lowered intake depends on whether you are a man or a woman. Women do not deplete glycogen as quickly as men do and therefore tend to respond better if carbs, and therefore insulin, are kept lower for longer periods. (Glycogen is basically carbohydrates that are stored in the liver and muscle tissue. Depleting these stores increases the use of fat for fuel.) This means that women should begin by restricting carbs to 30 grams per day or less for *13 consecutive days* in order to deplete glycogen and naturally inhibit their alpha receptors. Men, on the other hand, have an easier ride and deplete muscle glycogen at a much faster rate. Because of this, men usually do well with shorter periods of similar carb restriction (6 consecutive days). However, if you are a man and have a significant amount of fat to lose, I recommend starting with 13 consecutive days before introducing a "refeed" day (or a period during the day when you eat your favorite foods). After four weeks you can try adding in an additional high-carb meal midweek (after your workout) and gauge the results.

A low-carb day does not mean that you can't eat any carbohydrate foods. After all, vegetables contain carbs, and eliminating those would be a bad idea. You just have to be more selective. Following these rules will make things easy:

1. **Do not eat processed or starch-based carbohydrate foods.** This includes all breads (whole-wheat or otherwise), pastas, rice (white and brown), potatoes, and yams, and anything made from corn. You may be thinking, "What the heck am I supposed to eat, then?" Don't worry; I will get to that in a moment.

2. **Do not drink any beverages that contain sugar or high-fructose corn syrup.** Remember, the goal with carb fasting is to minimize blood sugar spikes and control insulin. Fruit juice and soft drinks will send your blood sugar soaring. I am not a big fan of artificial sweeteners either, but if you must have diet soda, have it sparingly. Keep in mind that some studies have shown artificial sweeteners to be potent stimulators of appetite

and weight gain. Finally, if you are going to drink alcohol, adhere to the rules outlined in chapter 5.

3. **Reduce or eliminate fruit from your diet (at least for the time being).** When you eat fruit, fructose is shunted to the liver, where it is converted into glycogen. The pathway for conversion of fructose to body fat is surprisingly efficient when muscle and liver glycogen levels are full. If you do choose to eat fruit, do so on days when your total carbohydrate intake is low, and stick with low-sugar fruits such as small, dark berries. There is one fruit that I do recommend you eat (in moderation): avocado. This fruit is rich in essential fatty acids and has a positive impact on blood sugar, satiety, and insulin. For those who have a sweet tooth and are looking for a sugar substitute, choose stevia over agave, which is 90% fructose.

TEMPORARY CARBOHYDRATE DEPLETION: BENEFITS WHEN IT COMES TO FAT LOSS

1. Carb depletion empties your body's glycogen reserves. When liver and muscle glycogen levels are full, ingested carbohydrates "spill over" and are easily stored in fat cells. Depleting carbohydrates stops this from happening and drains your body's glycogen stores, allowing your body to use fat for fuel.
2. Depleting carbs lowers blood sugar and insulin, promoting a more efficient fat-burning environment.
3. Carb depletion can create a calorie deficit, which is necessary for losing body fat.

WHAT CAN I EAT?

Depending on where you live and how you have been raised, the three rules for following a low-carb diet will either be a breeze or the single biggest challenge you have ever faced. Experience has taught me that more often than not, it's the latter. Do not despair. The carbs will return, and in the meantime, there are many fantastic foods you can eat.

The foods listed in the foods chart on the following page are allowed during a fat-loss phase. I want you to stick to purely fibrous carbohydrates during the first two weeks. Legumes are higher in carbs but acceptable for some people because those carbs come from fiber content. I say "some" people because not everyone fares well eating legumes, due to their high lectin content. Lectins are carbohydrate-binding proteins that can wreak havoc in the digestive tract, making them very difficult to digest (hence the flatulence jokes). If you do choose to include legumes in your diet, preparation is ultimately important. This usually means using dried beans and a diligent soaking process to improve their digestibility (canned legumes contain more preservatives and are often exposed to BPA). If this is something you are prepared to do, you can choose from:

Black beans
Lentils
Pinto beans
Red beans

Note: I do eat edamame on occasion, but soybeans are something I generally avoid because of their estrogenic properties. Soybeans contain genistein and daidzein, which are phyto-estrogens (estrogens produced by plants). If consumed in large quantities, these may disrupt the body's endocrine systems. A recent Harvard study revealed a strong association between men's consumption of soy foods and decreased sperm counts. In addition, hexane, a byproduct of gasoline refining and a known neurotoxin, often is used in the production of processed

PROTEIN	FIBROUS VEGETABLES	FATS
Chicken (free-range when possible)	Alfalfa sprouts	Avocados
Cottage cheese	Artichoke hearts	Borage oil
Crab	Asparagus	Coconut oil
Beef, extra lean	Bamboo shoots	Fish oil
Buffalo, extra lean	Bean sprouts	Flaxseed: ground flaxseed and flax-seed oil
Eggs	Beets	
Haddock	Bok choy	
Halibut and tilapia	Broccoli	Grapeseed oil
Herring	Brussels sprouts	Olives and extra-virgin olive oil
Kefir	Cabbage	
Lobster	Carrots	Organic butter
Mackerel	Cauliflower	Organic peanut or almond butter*
Milk	Celery	
Nuts and seeds	Collard greens	Primrose oil
Pickerel	Cucumber	Raw nuts: almonds, cashews, and walnuts
Protein powders: whey and veg-etarian (must not contain artificial sweeteners and other junk)	Dandelion greens	
	Garlic	
	Green beans	Raw Seeds
	Kale	Whole eggs
	Kimchi (made from napa cabbage)	
Salmon (wild)	Kohlrabi	*Note: Avoid consum-ing nonorganic peanut butter, as it contains aflatoxin, a mold.
Sardines	Leeks	
Scallops	Lettuce	
Shrimp	Mushrooms	
Tempeh	Okra	
Tilapia	Onion	
Tofu	Parsley	
Tuna, canned light (packed in water)	Peas	
	Peppers	
Turkey (free-range when possible)	Radicchio	
	Radishes	
Yogurt	Rhubarb	
	Sauerkraut	
*Note: To avoid develop-ing a protein intolerance, always rotate your pro-tein selections and try to not eat the same protein source back to back. And always choose organic sources when possible.	Scallions	
	Sea vegetables (dulse, nori, kombu)	
	Spinach	
	Tomato	
	Zucchini	
	*Note: Small amounts of legumes can also be eaten but only after day 13.	

soybean food products (whenever possible choose 100% certi-fied organic soy products).

It is imperative that you consume a sufficient amount of fat during a low-carb phase. If fat intake is too low, your body will be forced to use protein for energy through a process known as *gluconeogenesis,* or glucose creation, which is not conducive to fat burning. Another problem with avoiding fats during a low-carb phase is cravings—they will drive you crazy! Keeping fat intake relatively high will help keep cravings at bay during the periods when your carb intake is low. For these reasons, it is important that you don't shy away from eating fat with your low-carb meals. For those who like to run the numbers, I rec-ommend that you eat half a gram of fat for every gram of pro-tein (this doesn't have to be exact, just make sure to have some fats with your protein).

Remember, unless you have hypothyroidism, saturated fat (found in meat, eggs, and dairy products) should *not* be avoided. There are hormonal benefits to consuming some satu-rated fat, and new research shows that eating foods high in this type of fat does not contribute to elevated cholesterol levels and heart disease (the evidence suggests that heart disease is linked to excessive inflammation caused by consuming processed, refined foods, not high cholesterol). Cholesterol is the build-ing block for sex hormones like testosterone, which contributes to optimal health and body composition. The only type of fat that should be avoided is trans fat. Trans fats have no health benefit whatsoever and consuming them will only increase your trouble spot fat deposits and harm your health. Trans fats are found in processed junk foods such as donuts, french fries, store-bought cookies and muffins, and potato and corn chips. These fats should only rarely (if ever) be consumed, even on a cheat day.

What about Calories?

I am a car guy, and I enjoy driving a nice ride. When it's time for me to get a new one, I always do a ton of research. Before I make my decision I consider many factors beyond price, including performance, ergonomics, and, of course, fuel economy. My present car has a US Environmental Protection Agency rating of 21 city and 28 highway miles per gallon. Given my driving habits, though, I rarely keep anywhere close to those numbers.

The way we burn calories is similarly variable, and there is no practical way to calculate with any degree of accuracy how many calories you require at any given moment. Precise calorie counting would make sense only if your body obtained the same amount of energy from 100 calories of protein as it does from 100 calories of carbohydrates—which it doesn't. Old-school dieticians will tell you to count every crumb you consume, but this is an oversimplification of a complex process. Make no mistake, calories do matter, but no convenient and reliable way of measuring them exists. A more pragmatic approach is to focus on the quality of calories and use the guidelines below to determine roughly the quantities of food you should be eating when you are carb fasting.

Women: each meal should consist of:
- 1 palm-sized portion of protein
- 1 fist-sized portion of vegetables
- 1 thumb-sized portion of fats

Men: each meal should consist of:
- 2 palm-sized portions of protein
- 2 fist-sized portions of vegetables
- 2 thumb-sized portions of fats

Use these guidelines as a starting point, and pay close attention to how your body responds. If you find yourself overly hungry or feeling very weak and lethargic, adjust the portions accordingly. You may be asking yourself, "When will I ever eat carbs again?" Just hold on and keep reading because I am about to show you where those fit into the picture.

WHAT CAN I DRINK?

Beer. I'm joking. Doubtlessly, you have heard it many times before, but it is worth repeating: water is the best possible beverage. Now, you don't need to carry around a 2-gallon jug everywhere you go. That would make long commutes almost impossible and is just weird. One of the main reasons you want to increase water intake on a fat-loss program is to optimize liver function. Your liver is responsible for nutrient breakdown, storage, and detoxification, and water is required for it to perform these tasks efficiently. I recommend drinking approximately half your body weight in ounces of water daily. Using this calculation, a 140-pound person would consume 70 ounces, or about 9 cups, per day. Increase the amount if you exercise in the heat or perspire heavily. You should also drink more water on cheat days. Finally, I also recommend squeezing fresh lemon or lime juice into your water. This will make it taste better, so it's easier to drink more water, and aid in the detox process.

What about Milk?

One of the more interesting developments in sports nutrition in the last few years has been the change in the dairy industry's marketing focus. It now has television commercials and print ads expounding the virtues of chocolate milk as a post-workout beverage.

Even some Internet fitness gurus have jumped on the bandwagon, supporting chocolate milk as a recovery drink. These gurus and the manufacturers are saying that chocolate milk has an ideal macronutrient ratio for post-recovery, that being an approximate 2:1 ratio of carbs to protein, with minimal calories from fat.

Now, if you just look at what they are basing their claims on, you will be hard-pressed to find any issues with it. After all, a low-fat, moderate-protein, high-carb beverage is generally ideal when it comes to a post-workout drink.

But if you dig a little deeper, you will soon discover why chocolate milk is actually a very poor choice, and that it may be making you sick, weak, and osteoporotic.

Here are the facts when it comes to milk, chocolate or otherwise:

- **Milk is very acidifying to the body.** Your body has a pH level that is regulated to stay between 6.8 and 7.4. When your body becomes too acidic (because of the overconsumption of high-acid-forming foods like dairy products, meats, and grains), it will look for ways to neutralize the high acid load by using a "base" or alkalizing substance, mainly calcium or glutamine. The problem is that the calcium is leached from your bones (making you prone to osteoporosis) and the glutamine is taken from your muscles (turning you into a "girly" man or woman). Both are equally bad.
- **Milk contains lactose.** Lactose is basically sugar, which will raise insulin levels. Now, raising insulin post-workout isn't necessarily a bad thing. The problem is that most people suffer from lactose intolerance to some degree. Yes, this means that even though you may not be officially lactose intolerant, your body probably still doesn't deal well with the lactose. Mild allergic reactions to milk include inflammation, water retention, and mucous formation.

- **Milk can disrupt your endocrine system.** Dairy products that come from nonorganic sources may be chock-full of antibiotics, bovine growth hormones, and other wonderful hormonal disrupters that do nothing to make your body, including your bones, healthy. If you must drink milk (and I have no idea as to why that would be), it is advisable that your milk comes only from cows that are grass-fed and hormone-free. (Same goes for the beef you eat.)

I am far from being a lone wolf on this issue. Much has been written about this topic, and there are several documentaries and news reports on the subject. The problem is that these reports are often stifled in mainstream media. To lose trouble spot fat, forgo nonorganic dairy entirely and stick to fermented options such as kefir and unsweetened yogurt.

HOW TO BINGE FOR FASTER FAT LOSS

Hallelujah, here come the carbs! By now you know that carb restriction is necessary for mobilizing trouble spot fat. But the effect of carb fasting is only temporary. If carbs and calories are restricted for too long, your body will fight back by increasing appetite, slowing metabolism, lowering testosterone, increasing cortisol and fat-storing hormones, and decreasing fat-burning hormones. This is, of course, a very bad thing, and one of the reasons very-low-calorie diets have a high rate of failure.

Unfortunately, eating a high-calorie diet for an extended period is not the answer either (sorry). However, having *periodic* days of increased calories (in particular, carbohydrate calories) after a period of low calories/low carbohydrates will temporarily reverse all the negative adaptations and increase metabolism, decrease fat-storing hormones, and increase fat-burning, muscle-building hormones.

That is a simplistic explanation of a complex series of processes occurring inside your body, but it paves the way to my point, which is this: You *must* "cheat" on your diet.

Yes, periodic diet breaks, "refeed" days or "cheats," can (and should) be a part of your life, as they can help speed up the fat-loss process and make life *much* more enjoyable.

Now, before you run off to Ben & Jerry's for an ice cream orgy, you need to know some guidelines:

1. **You must be in a calorie deficit most of the time** for the cheat to work (and if you ever want to lose your trouble spot fat).

2. **There are three types of cheats:** cheat meals, cheat windows, and cheat days. I don't recommend an entire day of free eating. You know the old saying "Give someone an inch and they'll take a mile"? Well, that certainly applies here. Quite often, if a person is told they can eat whatever they want for an entire day, they will start jamming every food they have ever craved into their mouths, starting at six o'clock in the morning and not stopping until they go to bed (which will be very late, just so they can cram in some more junk). This is not only stupid, it will also cause problems. Instead, allow yourself a cheat window. For example, allow yourself three hours of your cheat day to indulge and then stop the madness.

3. **Always start and end the day with protein.** This should remain consistent throughout the week. No deviations here, please.

4. **Don't eat high-carbohydrate foods plus high-fat foods.** This is the worst combination. I'd prefer that you have a high-carbohydrate cheat rather than a high-fat cheat. If you want to do a high-fat cheat, then don't go crazy with the carbs.

5. **Choose "better" carbohydrate foods**, even on a cheat day. Glucose and *glucose polymers* (a type of processed carbohydrate) do a much better job at restoring glycogen levels than do sucrose or fructose. Foods that are high in glucose include pasta, whole-grain bread and cereals, potatoes, legumes, grapes, and squash. Simple, refined sugar in the form of cakes, candies, and so on offer no nutritional benefit whatsoever. In fact, research has shown that consuming refined sugar decreases immune system function, stimulates appetite through a reduction in leptin, can cause cellular damage, and may even fuel the development of cancer cells. If you are craving these foods and are intent on consuming them, you may do so on your cheat day, but I want you to pay attention to how your body feels the next day. Personally, consuming large amounts of refined sugar does not agree with me and often causes stomach upset and excessive feelings of lethargy the next day (the majority of my clients have reported this also). For this reason I prefer to cheat using other foods instead. The only way you will know what works best for you is to experiment with eating different foods and to notice how your body responds.

   Note: In the past few years, I have seen an increase in the incidence of gluten intolerance. This condition may present itself in various symptoms, including:

Digestive symptoms:
- Frequent gas or bloating
- Irritable bowel syndrome or acid reflux
- Daily diarrhea or chronic constipation

Neurologic and skeletal symptoms:
- Migraine or headaches
- Joint pain
- Brain fog

Hormonal and immune symptoms:
- Depression or anxiety
- Chronic fatigue
- Eczema or acne

If you even suspect that you may be suffering from gluten intolerance, I strongly recommend removing all carbohydrate foods that contain gluten. These include wheat, rye, barley, spelt, kamut, and oats contaminated with gluten during processing. In their place you can eat gluten-free carbs, such as quinoa, gluten free oats, buckwheat, rice, potatoes, and sorghum.

6. **Avoid drinking alcohol with high-fat meals.** Otherwise this is a recipe for more fat no matter what. If you want to have a drink, have it with vegetables or protein instead. High-fructose corn syrup should also be avoided in general, but especially in combination with alcohol.

7. **If you're a man, see if you benefit from having two cheats per 14-day cycle** (for example, on day 7 *and* day 14). The best way to figure out if you would is to start with one cheat period, and after four weeks introduce a second cheat mid-cycle. If you find that this stalls progress, you can always switch back. No two bodies respond exactly the same, and that's why there is a need for flexibility with any intelligent program.

8. **Don't have two cheat days back to back.** Two full days of cheating in a row can cause you to spin out of control and set you back on a path of poor eating. For men,

always separate them by four to six days; for women, over double that length of time—the cheat day should be after day 13. For example, a man could have a cheat meal on Saturday while out at a restaurant with friends and then have a treat again on the following Friday. A woman should spread it out by an extra week because women deplete muscle glycogen at a slower rate than men.

9. **Use supplements to mitigate insulin response.** The average person cheats with high-carbohydrate foods, not high-fat foods. Foods like bread and milk and chocolate cake tend to be more popular as cheat meals than a fatty pork chop, for example. If this describes you, then try supplementing with 3 grams (½ teaspoon) of cinnamon, 2 grams of fish oil, and 1 cup of green tea, taken separately, twice during your cheat day to keep insulin under control.

10. **Skip breakfast the day after a cheat day.** The morning after a cheat day, I often wake up only to find that I am not at all hungry. If this happens to you, feel free to forgo breakfast and simply resume your normal eating pattern at lunchtime. It can take a considerable amount of time for your body to digest and process the excess calories consumed on a cheat day, and there is no risk of muscle loss from periodic fasting.

    Don't be surprised to see, when you stand on the scale the day following a cheat, that you have gained a few pounds. This is normal, and it is *not* due to fat. Your body will retain a bit of water, but some of it will be in your muscles, potentially making you look even better!

11. **Exercise the evening before or the morning of your cheat day whenever possible.** You can do cardio or weights (no intervals or super-heavy training in a

carb-depleted state, please). Exercising at this time depletes glycogen and activates GLUT4, a glucose transporter that helps shuttle nutrients to your muscles instead of to your fat cells. Resistance exercise works best, as it increases the number of GLUT4 receptors per cell while simultaneously increasing their receptivity.

12. **Take advantage of the excellent opportunity the day after a high-carbohydrate cheat day to build more muscle.** Your body's muscle-building hormones will be amped up on that day, and you will experience some tremendous "pumps." This is a good day to perform heavy-weight training or high intensity interval training (HIIT).

YOU'VE GOT QUESTIONS? I'VE GOT ANSWERS!

Q: How often should I eat?

A: Perhaps the biggest nutrition myth to be debunked in recent times is that of high meal frequency being superior to low meal frequency for fat loss, muscle building, and so on. Here is what I have observed: during a fat-loss phase, a low meal frequency works best. This is for two reasons.

First, because you will be eating fewer calories, it simply may not be practical to be eating five or six times per day. For example, if you need to eat 1400 calories in order to be in a calorie deficit and lose fat, spreading those calories out over five meals will leave you eating portions so small that you may never feel satisfied. The easiest way to reduce calories is to decrease the number of times you eat, not increase it.

Second, skipping meals during a fat-loss phase may be beneficial from a hormonal standpoint. During periods of fasting, the catabolic hormones cortisol and adrenaline are elevated, creating an excellent environment for fat burning, especially when you train during this period. This builds the case for reducing meal frequency when trying to lose body fat. This is not to say that you can't lose fat eating five or six small "meals" per day. You simply have to experiment to find out what works best for you. It has been my experience that in order to lose trouble spot fat, one has to get comfortable with being hungry several days per week. This feeling of hunger will abate somewhat over time, but be prepared for a little discomfort. I never said this was going to be easy!

Q: Can I skip breakfast?
A: It's a tough question. I've experimented with this extensively, and for me the answer is no. I found that whenever I skipped breakfast, unless it's after a cheat day, I simply felt like complete dog crap the rest of the day. I also felt the same way when I ate lots of carbs for breakfast. This does not mean that you will have the same result. I have known many people who prefer to skip breakfast and are able to maintain an excellent physique. The choice is yours. Try experimenting with your meal frequency. Here are some options.

FOUR MEALS PER DAY	THREE MEALS PER DAY	TWO MEALS PER DAY
• 6 a.m.: Breakfast	• 12 p.m.: Lunch	• 12 p.m. Lunch or 6 p.m. Dinner
• 12 p.m.: Lunch	• 6 p.m.: Dinner	• Post-workout recovery beverage
• 5 p.m.: Dinner	• Post-workout recovery beverage	
• Post-workout recovery beverage		

Q: Do I need to count calories?
A: The number one factor in losing body fat is calorie balance. What does this mean? It means that calories count. In order for your body to tap into stored body fat, one of two things must happen: you must reduce calorie intake, or increase calorie

expenditure through exercise. Or do both. No amount of food combining, fasting, supplementation, or protein and carb manipulation can substitute for this. In all things, calorie balance reigns supreme. Every diet book is predicated on this one simple fact (although the bestselling ones are good at disguising it in order to trick people into thinking something else is going on). It is critically important that you accept this fact. Most people tend to grossly *underestimate* the amount of calories they are eating and *overestimate* the number of calories they are burning through exercise. There is one very important point I would like to stress again: not all calories are created equal. Consuming 2000 calories per day of candy bars and potato chips will produce vastly different results than consuming 2000 calories of protein, vegetables, and essential fatty acids. This is mainly because of the beneficial effects of protein in terms of satiety and its thermogenic properties, and the nutritional value of whole foods.

Those people who are interested in building muscle, take note: you simply will not build any appreciable muscle mass unless you have sufficient food energy coming in. I guess this is a long-winded way of saying yes, you should have a very good idea of approximately how many calories you are consuming each day. I say "approximately" because you don't need to be exact. However, once you have reached your goal, you will have a good handle on how your body responds to the different eating and exercise strategies outlined in this book, and you will be able to eat more intuitively. You can try to do this without counting calories, but keep in mind that when it comes to producing a predictable result, it is always best to operate using real data and not guessing.

Here's a simple formula for calculating the daily calories required on a fat-loss program:

Body weight in pounds × 10 kcal = daily calorie intake

Now, this does not mean that you need to consume that precise amount of calories—keep in mind that your calorie intake will likely fluctuate, unless you eat the same exact things every day. Just try to keep the number to within 10% of the calculation, whether over or under.

Fat-Loss Calorie Guide

BODY WEIGHT	DAILY CALORIE INTAKE (-/+ 10% RANGE)
100 lb	1000 kcal (900–1100)
150 lb	1500 kcal (1350–1650)
200 lb	2000 kcal (1800–2200)
250 lb	2500 kcal (2250–2750)
300 lb	3000 kcal (2700–3300)

Remember to completely disregard your calorie-counting obsession on your high-carb days! If you still feel the need to track your calories, you may want to check out the free service offered at www.fitday.com.

Q: Are nuts okay? Aren't they high in fat and calories?
A: Yes, yes, and yes. *Raw* nuts and seeds are fantastic, but you have to be careful to not overconsume—it is very easy to slam back 500 calories in very little time. Do that two or three times in a day and watch your fat loss stall right out.

Q: How much protein should I eat?
A: Aim to get at least 0.75 to 1 gram of protein for every pound of body weight each weekday. This amount would be lower if you were a person who didn't exercise. Exercise increases the rate of protein turnover in your body, and protein is needed to facilitate tissue repair. You can eat less protein on your cheat

day, as the increased carbohydrates will have a protein-sparing effect. In other words, when you increase carbs, you won't need as much protein to fuel your body's demand for energy.

Q: Can I really eat anything I want on my cheat day?
A: Whenever I am asked this question, I know I am dealing with someone who doesn't completely get it. It's almost as though they see their body as a separate entity from themselves and view the fat-loss process as some kind of game. The short answer to this query is yes, but I really have to question why anybody would want to eat pure poisonous crap that can severely disrupt the metabolic and endocrine systems for several days. I prefer people to stick to high-carbohydrate, *real* food on their cheat day. This does include foods such as bread, pizza, and ice cream. Having a meal at your favorite restaurant is better than binging on packaged foods from the local convenience store. Foods full of artificial sweeteners, hydrogenated oils, and other garbage are always best avoided.

Q: Won't eating a low-carb diet cause muscle loss?
A: Whenever you limit calories, you run the risk of muscle loss. After all, dieting is a *catabolic* event. But it is the reduction in calories, and not the reduction of carbohydrates, that causes this. The only way to prevent muscle breakdown during periods of calorie restriction is by maintaining your protein requirements in conjunction with resistance training. Changing from using challenging weights and low reps to doing high reps with light weights is a mistake and usually results in muscle loss. Excessive high-intensity cardio while on a reduced-calorie diet will have the same result. The exercise programs described in this book are specifically timed to minimize any chance of muscle loss.

Q: How will I know if I have depleted glycogen and am ready for a cheat day?
A: The easiest way to tell is by gauging how you feel when performing high-intensity intervals. For most people, performing high-intensity interval training is best done in the day or two following a cheat. If you feel like total crap during your high-intensity training and are feeling noticeably weaker, it is time to replenish those glycogen levels.

Q: How long can I stay on this program?
A: I recommend that you follow the fat-loss strategy for a maximum of four to six weeks at a time. After each phase, it is advisable to switch to a muscle-building program as described in Part 4, "Your Body Plus the Muscle," and return to the fat-loss program if you regain the body fat.

Q: What should I do if the fat isn't coming off fast enough?
A: When talking about fat loss, it is important to understand what constitutes "fast." Sometimes a person gets upset because they have lost "only" 5 pounds after a month. Unfortunately, TV shows like *The Biggest Loser* have conditioned people to believe that weekly double-digit body fat reductions are the norm. They are not. This happens only with obese individuals, not with people who are trying to shed the last inch from around their belly button. That being said, if your fat loss stalls out, you need to change your approach. When you stall, try incorporating one 24-hour fasting period into your midweek schedule. This practice is known as intermittent fasting and simply means forgoing any food or liquid food energy for a given period (you can still consume beverages that don't have calories, such as tea, water, and—my fave—black coffee). Fasting is dead simple. For example, let's say you choose Monday as your day to fast. On Sunday you would consume your last meal at six o'clock in

the evening, and you then would not eat again until six o'clock on Monday evening. I also recommend trying, whenever possible, to perform an exercise session while in this fasted state, as this can amplify the fat-burning effect.

The ideal day to fast is the day following your cheat period. On this day, your glycogen levels will be full, and you may find that you're not that hungry anyway (because of the large number of calories consumed the day before). Fasting on this day actually makes the whole process a lot less painful. In fact, many people find it quite liberating to not have to eat the day after consuming a considerable number of calories and carbs. If you find yourself feeling overwhelmed with hunger during your fasting day, try consuming 5 to 10 grams of branched-chain amino acids (BCAAs) every four hours or so (see chapter 9 for more on this supplement). This will help curb your hunger pangs and eliminate any chance of muscle loss during your fasting period.

8

The Adrenaline Protocols

Exercise for Maximum Fat Loss

In this chapter you'll learn everything you need to know about exercising for maximum fat loss. During this portion of the program, I want you to remain focused on one thing and one thing only: losing trouble spot fat. I tell you this to steer you away from the all-too-common mistake of pursuing mutually exclusive goals. Although the promise of building muscle while losing fat sounds enticing, it is completely empty. The body can adapt maximally in only one direction or another. These goals are on opposite ends of the calorie spectrum—muscle building is an anabolic process that requires a calorie surplus, whereas fat loss is a catabolic process that requires a calorie deficit.

Early on in my fitness career, I spent some time modeling for fitness publications. Being exposed to this industry allowed me to gather some interesting insight into the world of fitness models. One thing I discovered was that all the male models were much smaller in person than they looked in their pictures. In fact, at 6 feet and 200 pounds, I was considered to be too big by many publications. I also discovered that the trick to looking great on the beach or in photos is to diet down and lose as much fat as possible first, and then shift focus by changing the program in order to gain some more muscle over a week or two. This creates a very tight-looking, visually impressive physique.

In chapter 3, I explained the fat-loss process and in chapter 4 the important role the catecholamines (adrenaline and noradrenaline) play in losing trouble spot fat. You will also recall that the hormonal response to exercise is amplified when the intensity of effort is increased. To that end, I have provided you with three resistance training protocols to choose from, and a cardio protocol that describes five options for that portion of your fat-burning workout. Most of the exercises in the protocols use free weights, body weight, or other portable gym equipment, not weight machines. I designed the workouts this way so they would be accessible to people who don't necessarily go to the gym (though you can certainly do these workouts there too) but who have the equipment and like to work out at home.

Keep in mind that the protocols will work for a period of time. Like all exercise programs, progressions are required to prevent stagnation. When it comes to exercise, I always prefer to do the least amount of activity that produces the greatest result. More volume or intensity of exercise does not necessarily produce better results. Sometimes all you get from doing more is injured, so please take heed.

While researching this program I found that the body responds better to certain types of exercise depending on the type of diet being followed. For example, on days that calorie and carbohydrate intake are low, it is best to use moderate to low-intensity exercise with longer duration. Conversely, on days after calories and carbohydrates are increased, it is best to crank up the intensity a notch and really test your limits. With this in mind, let's take a look at the protocols.

COMPLICATE TO PROFIT, SIMPLIFY FOR RESULTS

It seems like every time I turn on the television, there's a new exercise, supplement, or nutrition technique being touted as "the answer" to losing body fat. Oftentimes, companies use complicated terms to describe how their system or product is different from the others out there. The truth is, the basic fundamentals of human movement haven't changed much in some 2000 years, and when it comes to losing fat, it is best to keep things simple.

TRAIN BY YOUR GOAL, NOT BY YOUR GENDER

One common mistake that I often see personal trainers making has to do with how they design workouts for men and women, allowing a person's gender, rather than goal, dictate the exercise program. If you were to examine the muscle fibers of a man and a woman under a microscope, you would find that they are virtually identical. What does differ is the hormone levels of the body where they reside. Women have substantially lower levels of testosterone. In fact, most men have 10 times (or more) the amount of testosterone women possess. But if you are a man and you want to lose fat, you could easily get great results using a program that is very similar to a woman who shares the same goal. Of course, the weights used would differ proportionate to strength, but the actual exercises would be the same.

What this means is that, regardless of your sex, your goal should *always* dictate the training program. The only legitimate discrepancy I have observed when it comes to the design of male and female training programs is exercise frequency—women tend to have greater recovery ability and benefit from a higher training frequency (likely because women's bodies deplete glycogen at a slower rate than men's). With that in mind, let's take a look at the different movements you will be required to perform.

THE FIVE PRIMARY MOVEMENTS FOR FAT LOSS

Only five resistance-training movements are required for eliminating trouble spot fat: squatting, pushing, pulling, lunging, and total body. When you build your workout around these primary movements, you can be assured that you are building a structurally balanced body. You will also look less like the meathead at your local gym whose body resembles a light bulb because of an aversion to leg training.

The five primary movements are guaranteed to boost your metabolism, build and maintain muscle mass, and help you lose body fat in the fastest time possible. Note that these are specific *movements*, not exercises. There are many different exercises within each category of movement, and even when you are following the protocols, you can substitute an exercise with a similar one that works the same muscles to add variety to your workouts.

Here are the details of the five primary movements, starting with the most important one of them all:

1. **Squat movements.** These could range from a barbell squat to a dumbbell squat, or could be any variation of the dead lift. Squat movements involve a significant amount of muscle mass, which is one of the keys to burning a lot of calories.
2. **Pushing movements.** Any type of push-up or dumbbell press or bench press, or even a standing shoulder press.
3. **Pulling movements.** Any type of row or pull-up and may include dumbbell rows, seated rows, chin-ups, or lat pull-downs.

4. **Lunging and single-leg movements.** These could be any movement that works one leg at a time, including a dumbbell lunge or split squat, reverse lunge or single-leg squat, one-leg lying hip extension, or even a one-leg hamstring curl.

5. **Total body movement.** This could be any sort of total body movement, such as a squat press, power clean, mountain climber, stability ball rollout, wood chop, burpee, or knee tuck on a stability ball. The only prerequisite is that the movement incorporate both the upper and lower body simultaneously.

THE GANGSTER TRIO: FAT-LOSS PROTOCOLS

The three fat-loss protocols are designed to increase in difficulty as you move from Protocol 1 through 3. In the spirit of achieving the best result with the least possible effort, I recommend that you start with Protocol 1. If you find that this is too easy or if it stops producing results, proceed to the next protocol.

Just one more thing: before you get started, you'll need to understand some basic terminology. I use a scale known as the rating of perceived exertion, or RPE, to explain how hard you are supposed to be working. I prefer using the RPE scale as opposed to target heart rate because substances such as caffeine, synephrine, and ephedrine stimulate beta receptors and the sympathetic nervous system, resulting in an increase in heart rate, giving a false representation of how hard you are actually working. I discuss these types of stimulants in chapter 9, but for now just understand that heart rate is an unreliable method of gauging effort.

The RPE scale, used to measure the intensity of your exercise, ranges from 0 to 10. The numbers relate to phrases that are used to rate how easy or difficult you find an activity. For example, 0 (nothing at all) is how you feel when sitting in a chair, whereas 10 (very, very heavy) is how you feel at the end of an extremely difficult bout of exercise. (When it feels like your heart is about to burst out of your chest!)

RPE SCALE

0	Nothing at all
0.5	Just noticeable
1	Very light
2	Light
3	Moderate
4	Somewhat heavy
5	Heavy
6	
7	Very heavy
8	
9	
10	Very, very heavy

© Gunnar Borg, 1970, 1985, 1994, 1998

SPECIAL NOTE

It is very important for you to train intelligently and not overdo things. Consider these eight points before beginning this (or any other) exercise program:

1. **If you are not sure how to perform the exercise properly, don't do it.** Always get personal instruction from a certified trainer.
2. **Stop if you feel pain.** Yes, there will be some discomfort, but you should know the difference between discomfort and pain from an injury. There are always plenty of alternative exercises for every movement.

3. **Start with lighter weights than you think you can handle.** In the first week, err on the side of caution by using lighter weights and doing fewer sets.

4. **Always put safety first.** Use a spotter if you are training with heavy weights. If you train alone at home, do *not* train to failure.

5. **Always wear good-quality running shoes.** If you perform intervals outdoors, choose a safe running surface (grass or track, rather than pavement). If you use a treadmill, be sure to operate it safely.

6. **Always adhere to the recommendations in this book.** Do *not* do interval training more than four times per week. This *will* lead to overtraining and injury.

7. **Never skip the warm-up. Ever.** This is critical to staying injury-free.

8. **Always check with your doctor before starting any new exercise or diet program.**

GETTING STARTED

Your body's ability to utilize fat for fuel is optimized during periods when carbohydrate intake is low. The low carbohydrate and insulin levels will allow for a natural inhibition of the alpha receptors, resulting in the release of trouble spot fat.

Start with the Least

Start with the least amount of exercise (such as Protocol 1, three times per week). As you progress you can start including extra cardio sessions on your off days from lifting. Approach cardio as if you were adding spices to a dish—start with a small amount and add more as required. Remember that during this fat-loss phase you will be eating fewer calories and carbohydrates and will not feel like the Energizer Bunny. Running yourself down with excessive high-intensity exercise will only lead to muscle loss and injury. These activities tap into the anaerobic energy–production pathway, which is fueled by glucose. If you don't have sufficient carbohydrate intake, your body will eventually break down muscle tissue through gluconeogenesis to provide the glucose necessary to fuel high-intensity activity. This is why it is important to include a minimum of one high-carb eating period every 14 days.

PROTOCOL 1: WEIGHTS PLUS CARDIO SUPERSETS

This protocol is best performed three times per week on non-consecutive days. You can perform this at any time during the day, and you should experiment with finding what time works best for you. This protocol combines interval weight training and steady-state cardio. Here is how it is done.

Step 1. Perform a 5-to-10-minute dynamic warm-up (see the protocol pages). Warming up is critical, as it prepares your muscles, joints, and ligaments for movement while simultaneously helping to lower insulin for better fat-burning effect.

Step 2. Perform a total body, resistance-training workout. This workout incorporates three rounds of four supersets (two exercises performed back to back with minimal rest in between). Exercises alternate between upper-body and lower-body movements.

In terms of repetitions, because this is a fat-loss phase, the goal is to burn calories, deplete glycogen, and fatigue muscle tissue. This is not the time to be thinking about setting personal bests in your 1 rep max. One mistake people often make is based on the commonly held belief that high reps are better for fat burning. It is not necessarily the amount of weight you use, or the number of repetitions performed, that enhances fat burning but the intensity of effort produced by the workout.

The goal is to create muscular fatigue through short rest intervals, which has a powerful hormonal and metabolic effect. Just keep in mind that the number of repetitions performed will have an influence on the training effect.

For example, if your primary goal is to increase strength, speed, and power, spend the majority of your total exercise volume* lifting heavy weights in the 1 to 6 rep range. If endurance is your goal, you would be better served by lifting in the 15 to 25 rep range for most of your workout. If fat loss is what you are after, lifting in the range of 7 to 15 reps works very well. And finally, if bigger muscles are all you desire, you would be well served spending time lifting in *all* the above ranges, as they tap into different muscle fibers (I show you a very cool way of doing this in chapter 10).

All this is not meant to be absolute. There are benefits to including a variety of repetition ranges regardless of what your goal is, and your program can incorporate a percentage from each. The Training Goals chart on the following page can be used as a guideline for structuring your workouts based on your primary exercise goal.

WHAT MATTERS MOST

By now you know that what matters most for fat loss is overall calories burned, and this is a function of effort, not simply reps. You will see that in the fat-loss workouts, most exercises fall within the 8 to 15 rep range. If you are advanced, you could use slightly heavier weights and lift in the 6 to 10 range; if you are a newbie, feel free to lighten things up a tad and lift in the 12 to 20 range. Make sure you always use the *most weight possible while maintaining good form* for these exercises and increase the weight from week to week.

---

* Exercise volume refers to the total amount of time you spend exercising.

I designed these sample workouts for a fat-loss phase. Modify as you see fit by simply choosing one exercise for the upper body and one exercise for the lower body. Just try to keep with the general theme outlined below. You don't necessarily have to do the exercises in the order I've suggested, but it's imperative that you keep the rest periods to a minimum. The RPE during the weight-training intervals should be approximately 7 (very heavy). Once you have finished your supersets, complete 20 to 30 minutes of steady-state cardio (see page 151) at a RPE of approximately 3 to 4 (moderate to somewhat heavy).

Training Goals

EXERCISE VOLUME	REP RANGE
TO INCREASE STRENGTH	
80–100%	1–6
0–20%	7–15
0–10%	16+
TO BURN FAT	
0–15%	1–6
70–85%	7–15
0–15%	16+
TO BUILD MUSCLE	
0–30%	1–6
30–60%	7–15
0–30%	16+

Weights plus cardio supersets • PROTOCOLS

NOTE:

- Start every workout with the warm-up circuit.

- In Protocol 1, A1 and A2, B1 and B2, and so on, denote "super-sets," which are exercises performed back-to-back *without rest*. Rest for 45 seconds at the end of each superset before proceeding to the next superset and for two to three minutes at the end of each round of four supersets.

- The three-digit sequence beside each exercise represents the lifting tempo. Using squats as an example, "3-0-1" means that you should take 3 seconds to lower your body and without pausing push back up to the start position in 1 second. If you are performing a standing shoulder press with dumbbells, using a 3-2-1 tempo, you would start with both dumbbells above your head and lower them to shoulder height in 3 seconds, pause 2 seconds, and return to the starting position in 1 second.

- Finish each workout with stretching the tight muscle groups only.

PROTOCOL 1: RESISTANCE-TRAINING WORKOUT

WARM-UP CIRCUIT

- Begin with a 3-to-5-minute cardio warm-up of your choice (biking, running, skipping, etc.).
- Next, complete 2 rounds of each of the following:
  - Lying hip extension × 15 reps
  - Bird dog × 10 per side
  - Y squat × 10

	SUPERSETS	# REPS	TEMPO
A1	Split squat with dumbbells	10/side	2-1-1
A2	Flat bench dumbbell chest press	10–12	2-1-1
	REST 45 SECONDS		
B1	Step-up with dumbbells	15/side	2-0-1
B2	Dumbbell row	10–12	2-1-1
	REST 45 SECONDS		

C1	Standing shoulder press with dumbbells	10–12	2-1-1
C2	Dumbbell squat	15–20	2-1-1
	REST 45 SECONDS		
D1	Stability ball jackknife	15–20	1-1-1
D2	Side plank		30–60 seconds/side

REST 2–3 MINUTES BEFORE REPEATING SUPERSETS A
THROUGH D 2 MORE TIMES FOR A TOTAL OF 3 ROUNDS

Finish with 20 to 30 minutes of steady-state cardio (see page 151) at a RPE of approximately 3 to 4 (moderate to somewhat heavy), followed by stretching of all major muscle groups.

This protocol should be performed on 3 nonconsecutive days (e.g., Monday, Wednesday, and Friday). Don't forget to do your cardio on your off days (see Protocol 4).

PROTOCOL 2: WEIGHTS PLUS CARDIO CIRCUITS

This protocol takes things up a notch in terms of difficulty and is very effective for increasing the catecholamine response. With this protocol, we are going to add an additional exercise to each superset, thus changing it from a superset to a circuit. As with Protocol 1, you will perform this workout 3 nonconsecutive days per week (for example, Monday/Wednesday/Friday). The exercises in each circuit are performed back to back, without rest. Rest for one minute at the end of each circuit and perform each circuit two to three times. The weights used will be heavier, and reps will be lower and in the 6 to 10 range. Feel free to modify the sample workouts as you like by substituting similar exercises (just try to keep with the general themes). For example, you might try a chin-up instead of a pull-up, or a dumbbell dead lift for a more moderate version of the dead lift using a barbell. The RPE during the weight-training circuits should be approximately 7 (very heavy). Once you have finished your circuits, complete 20 minutes of steady-state cardio (see page 151) at a RPE of approximately 3 to 4 (moderate to somewhat heavy).

Option 1

WARM-UP CIRCUIT

- Begin with a 3-to-5-minute cardio warm-up of your choice (biking, running, skipping, etc.).
- Next, complete 2 rounds of each of the following:
  - Lying hip extension × 15 reps
  - Bird dog × 10 per side
  - Y squat × 10

	CIRCUITS	# REPS	TEMPO
A1	Barbell dead lift	8-10	3-0-1
A2	Pull-up	6–8	2-0-1
A3	Triceps dip *or* close-grip push-up	8-10	2-0-1
	REST 1 MINUTE. REPEAT 2 MORE TIMES FOR A TOTAL OF 3 CIRCUITS		
B1	Barbell squat	8-10	3-0-1
B2	Standing shoulder press (dumbbells or barbell)	8-10	2-0-1
B3	Dumbbell row	8-10/side	2-0-1
	REST 1 MINUTE. REPEAT 2 MORE TIMES FOR A TOTAL OF 3 CIRCUITS		
C1	Lunge with dumbbells	8-10	2-0-1
C2	Flat bench dumbbell chest press	8-10	2-0-1
C3	Inverted row	8-10	2-0-1
	REST 1 MINUTE. REPEAT 2 MORE TIMES FOR A TOTAL OF 3 CIRCUITS		

Finish with 20 to 30 minutes of steady-state cardio (see page 151) at a RPE of approximately 3 to 4 (moderate to somewhat heavy), followed by stretching of all major muscle groups.

Option 2

If you are training at a public gym, it can sometimes be difficult to perform three different exercises in a row without ticking off other members for making them wait to use the equipment. If that is the case, you may want to try incorporating a non–weight-training exercise into the mix. See page 148 for a list of active rest options. Start with the warm-up circuit and proceed with the workout as follows:

	CIRCUITS WITH ACTIVE REST	# REPS	TEMPO
A1	Barbell dead lift *or* Barbell squat	8-10	2-0-1
A2	Triceps dip	8-10	2-0-1
A3	Active rest	20–30 seconds	
	REST 90 SECONDS. REPEAT 2 MORE TIMES FOR A TOTAL OF 3 CIRCUITS		
B1	Standing shoulder press (dumbbells or barbell)	8-10	3-0-1
B2	Lat pull-down *or* Dumbbell row	8-10 8-10/side	2-0-1 2-0-1
B3	Active rest	20–30 seconds	
	REST 90 SECONDS. REPEAT 2 MORE TIMES FOR A TOTAL OF 3 CIRCUITS		
C1	Flat bench dumbbell chest press	8-10	2-0-1
C2	Incline bench prone dumbbell row	8-10/side	2-0-1
C3	Active rest	20–30 seconds	
	REST 90 SECONDS. REPEAT 2 MORE TIMES FOR A TOTAL OF 3 CIRCUITS		

Finish with 20 to 30 minutes of steady-state cardio (see page 151) at a RPE of approximately 3 to 4 (moderate to somewhat heavy), followed by stretching of all major muscle groups.

ACTIVE REST EXERCISE OPTIONS

Battle rope
Bike or elliptical sprints
Burpees
High knees
Jumping with knee tucks
Medicine ball slams
Mountain climbers
Skipping rope
Treadmill sprints

PROTOCOL 3: METABOLIC TRAINING

Before you attempt this protocol, be aware that this one is not meant for beginners. Most people overestimate their athletic ability, and if you do that with the next workout, it may turn around and bite you in the ass! To do this protocol properly, you must have an excellent foundation of strength and the technical competence to execute each exercise with a high degree of proficiency. You also must have the ability to work through the pain and discomfort that is sure to happen whenever you perform compound exercises one after the other with no rest in between.

Another key difference with this protocol is that you will be performing not one but two bouts of exercise on certain days. "Two-a-days" are not for the faint of heart but few things work better for fat loss.

In this protocol, you'll perform the workout three non-consecutive days per week—for example, Monday (day 1)/ Wednesday (day 2)/Friday (day 3). On day 1 and day 3, in addition to your resistance training, you'll also perform an evening sprint workout (don't worry, it will take only 15 minutes and the results will be worth it). The exercises remain the same for each workout; however, you will change the weight and number of reps each day.

There is no rest between exercises A1 through A7, though you will rest 3 to 5 minutes at the end of each round. Use a controlled 3-0-1 tempo for each exercise and strive to maintain perfect form throughout.

Be sure to use a weight that is challenging for the number of repetitions done that day, and push yourself to improve each time you repeat the workout.

METABOLIC RESISTANCE TRAINING

MORNING/DAYTIME WORKOUT				
	EXERCISE (tempo 3-0-1)	MON # REPS	WED # REPS	FRI # REPS
A1	Barbell dead lift	4–6	10–12	15–20
A2	Pull-up *or* Lat pull-down	4–6	10–12	15–20
A3	Triceps dip *or* Close-grip push-up	4–6	10–12	15–20
A4	Split squat with dumbbells	4–6	10–12	15–20
A5	Standing shoulder press (dumbbells or barbell)	4–6	10–12	15–20
A6	Dumbbell row	4–6	10–12	15–20
A7	Side plank	30 seconds	60 seconds	90 seconds
REST 3–5 MINUTES. REPEAT 2 MORE TIMES FOR A TOTAL OF 3 CIRCUITS				
EVENING WORKOUT				
B1	200-meter sprint (approx. 30 seconds)	6 ×	—	6 ×
REST 2 MINUTES BETWEEN SPRINTS				

An important note on *progression*: your body will eventually adapt to any exercise stimulus, causing progress to slow to a halt. To avoid this, keep track of your sprint times and try to improve with each workout. Each week, the number of repetitions and sets, and the weight used, should increase while the rest period between circuits should decrease, to create a new stimulus for your body. Use the chart below to record and keep track of your sprint times, or create your own modeled on this one:

SPRINT TIME	
#1	#5
#2	#6
#3	#7
#4	#8

PROTOCOL 4: CARDIO WORKOUTS—STEADY-STATE AND HIIT

Cardiovascular training during a fat-loss phase is very much dependent on each trainee. Resistance training is not negotiable. It simply must be done if you want to look your best. Cardio, on the other hand, is dependent on the individual. It has been my experience that although many men can get great results without performing extra cardio sessions, very few women can say the same. In fact, in most cases, women *must* perform at least one or two cardio sessions a week on their off days in order to mobilize their trouble spot fat areas.

When it comes to losing body fat, cardio can be used to increase calorie expenditure, fat mobilization, and oxidation. The secret to making cardio work for you is to find your minimum effective dose. In other words, I want you to perform the minimum amount necessary to produce the best result. Doing too much will only run you down and cause you to lose more muscle than fat. The type of activity you choose can also impact your results. When choosing a cardio activity to lose fat, it is best to select one in which you are in a standing position (treadmill, stair climber, StepMill, running, etc.)—this is the position where the catecholamine release will be highest, resulting in the greatest release of fatty acids to be used for fuel.

STEADY-STATE CARDIO

This first option is very simple: perform 40 to 60 minutes of low-intensity, steady-state cardio, preferably in a fasted state and on non–weight-training days. For most people, this means first thing in the morning upon waking. I recommend having some caffeine, as well as 5 to 10 grams of branched-chain amino acids (BCAAs), before all fasted exercise sessions to prevent muscle loss and improve fat burning. Performing this protocol in a fasted state will not make or break the results, since exercise itself is very effective at lowering insulin. If you do not perform fasted, try to allow for two to three hours from the time of your last meal *or* simply extend the duration of exercise toward the 60-minute mark. Using the RPE scale on page 139, keep your RPE at approximately 3 to 4 (moderate to somewhat heavy) during this protocol. If you choose steady-state cardio, perform it no more than three times per week on days when your carbohydrate intake is low. This will lower insulin and allow for greater fat release.

Choose the type of exercise you're most comfortable with. For example, don't ride a bike if you prefer to walk. For steady-state cardio to work, you will need to spend some considerable time at it, and this just won't happen if you hate what you're doing. It is popular on the Internet these days to talk stink about steady-state cardio, and yet I have seen it produce remarkable results time and time again. Remember, these additional cardio sessions are to be performed on days when you do not train with weights.

HIGH-INTENSITY INTERVAL TRAINING (HIIT)

High-intensity interval training (or HIIT, as it is often called) is all the rage these days. The reason for its popularity is that the workouts are very short. You can work out hard or you can work out long, but it is very difficult to do both. Having experimented extensively with HIIT, I can say that it is not a panacea. Yes, it is very good for increasing anaerobic and aerobic capacity, and it is known to produce a greater calorie burn in the post-exercise period (the phenomenon known as EPOC, or excess post-exercise oxygen consumption). But one of the downsides of HIIT is the *potential* for muscle loss when performed in a carb-depleted state. In addition, not everybody has the capability to push themselves to the level of maximal intensity required for an effective HIIT workout. In the end what matters most when it comes to weight loss is muscle preservation and total calories burned during an exercise session. Whether you burn 300 calories in 10 minutes or in 30 minutes, the final result is pretty much the same.

One area where high intensity does make a difference is in catecholamine response and its effect on mobilizing trouble spot fat. Although all exercise increases the release of adrenaline and noradrenaline, their production is amplified when the intensity of effort is increased. The important thing to remember is that although HIIT will increase catecholamine output and subsequent release of fatty acids into the bloodstream, the exercise duration *must* be sufficient enough to allow those fatty acids to be fully taken up and utilized for energy.

If the duration is too short, these fatty acids may actually redeposit themselves elsewhere in the body through a process known as re-esterification. (Read on to see my recommendations for the duration of your HIIT.) I have seen the results of this: women whose breasts shrink while their thighs get bigger, which is enough to make just about any woman want to scream. The possibility of fatty acid re-esterification is the reason I always recommend performing some form of steady-state cardio exercise immediately following any interval-training workout, including after resistance-training workouts. I find this to be extremely effective for burning fat. In fact, it's the best fat-burning method I have ever used.

Women can (and should) perform HIIT more often than men. For most men, HIIT should be done sparingly, and sometimes not at all. If you are a guy who loves HIIT, it is better that you put it on the first and second days following a high-carb day. This is because performing HIIT when glycogen levels are depleted can cause muscle loss. As you know, glycogen is a combination of glucose and water, stored in the muscles and liver. Your body can hold only approximately 500 to 600 grams of glycogen at any one time. This equates to about two hours' worth of intense cardio (or less) for most men. What this means is that in order for men to prevent muscle loss and still work out hard the day following HIIT, they would need to ingest at least 600 grams of carbs. But consuming this amount of carbs will result in too much glucose and insulin for your body to deal with and will impede your fat-loss efforts. This is why I recommend having a source of protein or BCAAs before intense training in a carb-fasted state, as it helps prevent muscle catabolism.

Because women deplete muscle glycogen at a lower rate than men, they tend to respond better to more frequent HIIT sessions and can perform them more often. Again, I recommend starting with the least amount of work (one session per week on non–weight-training days) to see how your body responds. Don't perform HIIT the day before or the day after a heavy leg workout, as this can lead to overtraining.

HIIT cardio workouts can be performed in many ways. The word "interval" simply means a period of time. With high-intensity intervals you will be performing an interval of hard work followed by an interval of relatively easy work. My top three cardio machines in order of effectiveness and convenience are:

1. Treadmill
2. Stationary bike
3. Elliptical machine

The StepMill is also extremely effective, though most people do not have access to this machine.

For each level of HIIT, hop on the machine of your choosing and perform intervals as outlined. Adjust the speed and incline levels as needed.

Here are some examples of different types of intervals.

HIIT LEVEL 1

The work-to-rest ratio is 1:3. With this interval you will be working hard for 30 seconds and easy for 90 seconds over a period of time.

Warm up for 5 minutes (level 3.5)
Difficult for 30 seconds (level 7.0)
Easy for 90 seconds (level 3.5)
Difficult for 30 seconds (level 7.0)
Easy for 90 seconds (level 3.5)

Continue to alternate between intervals of difficult and easy for 20 to 30 minutes. Finish with 10 to 15 minutes of steady-state cardio (see page 151) at a RPE of approximately 3 to 4 (moderate to somewhat heavy), followed by stretching of the lower body.

This is a beginner's introduction to interval training and an excellent place to start. As soon as this becomes too easy, switch to performing Level 2.

HIIT LEVEL 2

The work-to-rest ratio is 1:2. With this interval you will be decreasing the rest and increasing the speed (and incline if using a treadmill). You will be required to work hard for 30 seconds and easy for 60 seconds.

Warm up for 5 minutes (level 3.5)
Difficult for 30 seconds (level 8.0)
Easy for 1 minute (level 5.0)
Difficult for 30 seconds (level 8.0)
Easy for 1 minute (level 5.0)

Continue to alternate between intervals of difficult and easy for 15 to 20 minutes. Finish with 15 minutes of steady-state cardio (see page 151) at a RPE of approximately 3 to 4 (moderate to somewhat heavy), followed by stretching of the lower body.

HIIT LEVEL 3

The work-to-rest ratio is 1:1. With this interval you will be decreasing the rest and increasing the speed even further. You will be required to work hard for 30 seconds and easy for 30 seconds.

Warm up for 5 minutes (level 3.5)
Difficult for 30 seconds (level 9.0)
Easy for 30 seconds (level 6.0)
Difficult for 30 seconds (level 9.0)
Easy for 30 seconds (level 6.0)

Continue to alternate between intervals of difficult and easy for 10 to 15 minutes. Finish with 20 to 30 minutes of steady-state cardio (see page 151) at a RPE of approximately 3 to 4 (moderate to somewhat heavy), followed by stretching of the lower body.

HIIT PYRAMIDS

Pyramids are a popular (and effective) way to add variety to your cardio workouts. Here is how they're done.

Warm up for 5 minutes
30 seconds difficult/30 seconds easy
1 minute difficult/1 minute easy
2 minutes difficult/2 minutes easy
4 minutes difficult/4 minutes easy
2 minutes difficult/2 minutes easy
1 minute difficult/1 minute easy
30 seconds difficult/30 seconds easy
Finish with a 10-minute cool-down

VARY THE INTENSITY AND DURATION

As with any type of workout, if you always do the same level of intensity and duration, you will eventually cease to progress. Always keep track of the workouts you perform, and keep trying to progress by changing up the variables.

SAMPLE WEEKLY WORKOUT CHART

MONDAY	Weights plus cardio
TUESDAY	Cardio only
WEDNESDAY	Weights plus cardio
THURSDAY	Cardio only
FRIDAY	Weights in a.m./Cardio in p.m.
SATURDAY	No training (cheat day)
SUNDAY	Interval cardio

RECOVER OR REGRESS

Although most people can appreciate the benefits that come from exercising, what most fail to realize is that it is often what we do after the workout that makes the biggest difference. Exercise is stimulus for change, but many of those changes happen while you are recovering and not during the exercise session itself. This means that proper recovery is an essential component of your workout routine and deserves as much attention as the exercises you perform. The muscle-recovery tips below will help ensure that you are getting the most benefit from the time you spend exercising.

Sleep

Your body does the majority of its restoration during sleep. Adequate sleep time varies for each person, but as a general rule you need between seven and eight hours of uninterrupted sleep each night. If this is not possible, try napping. A 30-minute power nap can be very effective at boosting recovery; it is best done about seven hours after waking. Make sure your sleep environment is dark and cool. As mentioned in chapter 1, try passion flower extract if you experience trouble falling asleep, and time-released melatonin for help staying asleep. If you have trouble waking, simply dip your feet in cold water!

Nutrition

Your post-workout meal is arguably the most important meal of the day and the one that is nonnegotiable. Favor a fast-digesting protein source (like whey isolate) with some quick-burning carbs (such as tropical fruits). Magnesium citrate is great for calming the nervous system after an intense workout. You can also blend up some greens and glutamine for a fantastic post-workout recovery drink.

Yoga

Yoga is an excellent recovery activity that should be performed once or twice a week. Yoga will improve your flexibility and recovery, and also enhance relaxation. There are hundreds of yoga poses, but here I have narrowed them down to just the bare essentials:

1. **Downward-facing dog**
   This pose strengthens the upper body, releases tension in the spine, and stretches out the back, calves, and backs of the thighs.
2. **Two-knee spinal twist**
   Performed on each side, this pose stretches and relieves tightness in the chest muscles, shoulders, upper and lower back, hips, and spine.
3. **Warrior II**
   This pose promotes balance in the hips, thighs, butt, and shoulders.

You can search the many yoga poses online at www.myyogaonline.com, or try a class with an experienced instructor.

Massage

Massage feels great and improves circulation. Self-massage is also beneficial. (Get your mind out of the gutter!) One session per week can work wonders for recovery.

Salt Bath

Bathing in Epsom salts is an excellent way to detoxify the body while simultaneously calming the nervous system, reducing swelling, and relaxing the muscles. Simply dissolve at least 2 cups into a bathtub of hot water and enjoy.

Contrast Shower

Alternating between bouts of very hot water and very cold water is an excellent way to improve recovery. (Just be sure to end with a bout of cold water if you need to stay alert. Ending with hot will have you dozing off quite nicely.) Try three minutes under the hot water followed by one minute using cold. Repeat three times and be sure to cover your whole body, including your head, with water.

Active Recovery

I have often found a light walk to be very therapeutic and excellent for clearing the mind and relaxing the body. Take some time to get outdoors for a walk, enjoying some fresh air and the sights and sounds of nature.

Time Off

Time off from exercise is an important part of the recovery process. Schedule periodic rest days (or even a week) to allow your body to repair and heal naturally. For some people, this can be one of the hardest things to do!

Soft-Tissue Work

Active Release Technique and other soft-tissue therapies are extremely effective for facilitating the healing process. One to two sessions per month works wonders at improving recovery and reducing injury.

Hydration

Being even slightly dehydrated will impair performance and impede metabolic functioning. Try consuming half your body weight in ounces of water each day to ensure proper hydration. Add a few squeezes of lemon juice (to help alkalize your body), and also a pinch of sea salt if you are a person who sweats a lot when you work out.

———

Incorporate any one of these techniques into your program, keeping in mind that varying your recovery techniques is as important as varying your training methods.

9

Supplements That Actually Work

I couldn't believe my eyes.

One inch. That's what the measuring tape said I had lost. In less than four weeks, my waist had dropped from 34 to 33 inches.

All because of one small addition to my supplement protocol.

What made the whole thing even stranger was that the "supplement" wasn't something you would ever think would increase fat loss . . .

The year was 1996, and I was preparing for a photo shoot for *Men's Exercise* magazine. I was 26 years old and fitness was my life. I ate, slept, and breathed bodybuilding. To become great at anything requires a significant amount of dedication, and bodybuilding is on the extreme end of the scale. I found myself immersed in the self-obsessed world of body transformation. For better or for worse, during this period, bodybuilding was my religion and, as such, *Muscle Media 2000* became my bible.

Muscle Media 2000 was the brain child of Bill Phillips, author of the *New York Times* bestseller *Body for Life*. At the time, *Muscle Media* magazine was known as the number one source of cutting-edge information about building muscle and losing body fat. In one issue, I was introduced to the concept of supplementing with essential fatty acids to lose midsection fat. The article claimed that adding essential fats to a person's diet would help improve insulin management and result in fat loss from the midsection.

And according to my measuring tape, it was right.

This was the first time I had ever used a supplement that produced such an undisputable result, and from then on I became very interested in learning everything possible about supplements and their effects on body composition.

PLAYING WITH FIRE

In the mid- to late 1990s, the supplement stack *du jour* was ephedrine, caffeine, and aspirin. It was cheap, easily available, and highly effective. The simple combination of 20 milligrams ephedrine, 200 milligrams caffeine, and 85 milligrams aspirin produced a profound thermogenic (and even mildly anticatabolic) response. This chemical cocktail worked to stimulate the body's beta receptors, resulting in significant fat loss.

But it was not a panacea. There were some serious side effects. The problem with ephedrine and other beta agonists is that there are beta receptors all over the various tissues of the body, including the heart. The use of such stimulants can result in dangerous cardiac abnormalities, and when excessive amounts are used, even death.

Because of these risks, I have since given up using ephedrine and fortunately have found that there are other supplements that can help with losing fat without the risks associated with this once popular concoction. This is not to say that ephedrine shouldn't be used by others, though. Chinese medicine often calls for the use of ephedrine as a decongestant, and I know many fitness competitors who cycle on and off ephedrine throughout the training year with no apparent ill effects. I myself have simply decided to avoid its use, as I find the side effects to be somewhat disturbing (heart palpitations are never much fun).

TIER 1 SUPPLEMENTS: THOSE YOU SHOULD BE USING

Losing body fat requires eating less food and a relatively simple diet. One of the strategies that works extremely well for me (and for my clients) is to embrace the idea that, when embarking on eating for extreme body transformation, boring is better.

By this I mean that it is a good idea, once you find four or five meals that are palatable and fit your diet criteria, to rotate through these same meals over and over (with the exception of your cheat days, when you should be eating other types of foods). This produces excellent results.

However, there is a potential problem with this strategy—the increased risk of developing nutrient deficiencies. Deficiencies in vitamins, minerals, and essential fatty acids can reduce insulin sensitivity and impair fat cell metabolism. At the same time, the need for nutrients increases as demands are imposed on your building, repairing, and recovery systems. When dieting, these demands are exacerbated because nutrients from food are diminished. Supplementation is necessary to address this issue. The following are the supplements I use and recommend. All of the supplements mentioned below can be found online or at your local nutrition store.*

---

* We are all unique and vary in our individual nutrient requirements. Always consult with your natural health practitioner for testing and dosing protocols.

1. **Fish oil.** This is perhaps the most studied supplement in history. Omega-3 fatty acids from fish play an important role in shedding trouble spot fat and a whole lot more. The beneficial components EPA (eicosapentaenoic acid) and DHA (docosahexaenoic acid) found in fish oil help reduce inflammation, boost immunity, and improve insulin sensitivity, among other things. Fish oil will also help increase blood flow to your trouble spot fat areas, and improved blood flow is crucial for mobilizing those hard-to-lose pounds. Look for an oil that is standardized to contain a minimum 2:1 ratio of EPA to DHA, and sourced from small fish like anchovies, sardines, and krill. The recommended dose is 6 to 20 grams per day. Stay on the low end of this scale if you are on blood-thinning meds, as fish oil has a blood-thinning effect.

2. **Probiotics.** Taking both *pre-* and *probiotics* can positively impact fat loss and mood. Your gut has trillions of bacterial cells that boost your immune system, fight off infections, influence fat absorption, and help with neurotransmitter production in the gut. These are the good bacteria. The bad bacteria do just the opposite. Unfortunately, many of us have more bad than good, and this can cause problems. Some simple ways to tip the scales in your favor include eating fermented foods (e.g., sauerkraut, kimchee, plain organic yogurt, kombucha, kefir), eliminating artificial sweeteners, and supplementing with probiotics. Prebiotics, the indigestible dietary fibers that probiotics use to flourish, grow, and proliferate, are also a wise addition. These can be found in the supplement inulin, as well as in FOS (fructooligosaccharides).

3. **Vitamin D and zinc.** Essential for life, vitamin D is

synthesized in the body as a result of sun exposure. It is vital for bone health, muscle mass, insulin management, immune function, brain health, disease prevention, and just about anything else you can think of. Most people living at northern latitudes are low in this, especially during the winter months. This makes supplementation essential. Checking vitamin D levels is simple, but it does require a blood test. Most people are in the range of 25 ng/ml, but you should work to bring this up to between 50 and 80 ng/ml. Generally, it takes about 15 minutes of exposure to the sun to make about 20,000 IUs of vitamin D. The efficiency of this production reduces with age, and by age 35, supplementation is generally required. I usually recommend between 1000 and 5000 IUs per day, and possibly more during the winter months. Increasing your vitamin D intake from food is also possible. The best sources are salmon, halibut, herring, tuna, mackerel, oysters, and shrimp. Shitake mushrooms are also a good source. But unless you are eating these foods daily and in sufficient amounts, you will have to use a supplement.

Zinc is also important. Found in virtually every tissue in the body, zinc is fundamental to hormone production and healthy endocrine function. If you are low in zinc, you will likely have low energy, poor immune function, chronic fatigue, and depressed anabolic hormone levels. Zinc deficiency is common, especially among vegetarians and those who exercise and sweat a lot. I take zinc twice daily, 75 milligrams with my first two meals of the day.

4. **B vitamins.** B vitamins are important for detoxification, decreasing estrogen load, metabolism, and energy production. They also make every other vitamin you

ingest work better. Because these vitamins are water soluble, I usually take two doses daily, one in the early morning and another in the late afternoon (avoid taking it in the late evening, as B vitamins may affect your ability to fall asleep). Don't be surprised by a change in the color of your urine.

5. **Whey protein and branched-chain amino acids (BCAAs).** These are two of my favorite supplements, and the ones I use most often. Whey protein is like fish oil in that there are so many studies proving its efficacy that stating them all would require a whole other chapter. Suffice to say that supplementing with whey protein is a fast way to increase your protein intake and reap its many benefits, including increased lean muscle tissue, decreased fat mass, improved immunity, and increased satiety. BCAAs (which are found in whey protein but also available separately in powder or capsule form) are very useful for building muscle, decreasing fat, increasing insulin sensitivity, and decreasing muscle soreness. Increased protein is necessary for avoiding losing muscle during periods of reduced calories and intense training.

6. **Greens+.** This is my favorite supplement of all time, and I rarely start a day without it. With the nutritional equivalent of six servings of organic vegetables, greens+ is a concentrated blend of vitamins, minerals, antioxidants, and green superfoods that promote an alkaline pH level in the body. Being too acidic can compromise immunity and deplete bone calcium and muscle glutamine levels, leading to osteoporosis and sarcopenia. I often double up on greens+ during periods of intense training by including a serving in my post-exercise protein recovery drink. This helps restore

an alkaline pH and makes me feel all warm and fuzzy inside knowing that I am giving my body something it really needs.

7. **Hydrochloric acid (HCl).** There is lots of talk about what foods we should eat, but we hear very little about what happens to those foods once they have been consumed. Digestion and assimilation of nutrients is the single most overlooked aspect of nutrition. The digestive fluid in your stomach contains sodium and potassium chloride, along with hydrochloric acid. People often lack HCl, and this impedes the absorption of nutrients and antioxidants, the breakdown of amino acids, and the activation of enzymes, all of which can impact your body composition. Your gut is your body's "second brain," and a deficiency in HCl can impact neurotransmitter efficiency and hormone production. If you think that because you have acid reflux you must have too much of the stuff already, think again. Health-care practitioners are often wrong when diagnosing hypochlorhydria, or low stomach acid. When HCl is too low, food isn't digested properly, and remnants can work their way back up the esophagus, causing a burning sensation. Taking antacids for this only worsens the problem. The solution is to *increase* stomach acid using supplemental HCl. The best way to tell if you have low stomach acid is to have yourself tested. A natural health-care practitioner will use the Heidelberg pH test, the most accurate way to gauge HCl insufficiency. Other common symptoms of low HCl include gas, bloating after eating, and undigested food in the stool. I use a digestive enzyme blend that contains HCl before every whole food meal and find this greatly improves my ability to digest food properly. (I don't take it before

drinking my protein shakes simply because the brand of protein I use has digestive enzymes included in the formulation.)

8. **Magnesium.** Along with vitamin D, magnesium is one of the most common nutrient deficiencies. A magnesium deficiency is associated with bone loss, osteoporosis, and even heart disease. People who are low in magnesium are usually low in vitamin D as well. Magnesium works to calm the nervous system, lowering stress and cortisol. I take 400 milligrams of magnesium glycinate before bed and after hard workouts. This is more easily absorbed by the body than the more common oxide form of magnesium that is often found in multivitamin formulations.

I consider the supplements listed above to be Tier 1 supplements. To enhance the fat-burning effect of your diet and exercise program, consider adding Tier 2 supplements, listed in the next section, to your regimen. The list may seem quite extensive, but remember that the use of these supplements is meant to be temporary and only during a fat-loss phase.

TIER 2 SUPPLEMENTS: FOR FAST FAT LOSS

1. **Caffeine.** On three occasions in my life I have dropped my body fat to below 6%, and each time, I used caffeine as part of my supplement arsenal. I discovered that 100 milligrams of caffeine right before my workout increased my motivation to exercise, and allowed me to exercise with greater focus and intensity and lose more body fat along the way. Caffeine can assist your workout in many ways, including by mobilizing fat stores; helping your muscles to access fat instead of carbs for energy; increasing testosterone, endurance, mental

focus, and exercise time to exhaustion; and relieving fatigue. Using caffeine pre-workout helps me lose more of the trouble spot fat that accumulates around my love handles—this is usually the most difficult spot for me to lose fat. Because caffeine raises blood sugar and cortisol, it should only be used pre-workout, so skip the post-workout Starbucks latte and opt for protein instead. But before you rush out and down 10 cups of coffee, listen up—caffeine is not without its side effects. Caffeine can temporarily elevate blood pressure and heart rate, but this effect is less pronounced in those who consume it on a regular basis. In addition, caffeine can induce blood sugar fluctuations, so keep this in mind if you have health issues related to blood sugar, such as diabetes. Since caffeine may interact with certain medications, always check with your doctor before introducing it into your diet. Finally, when choosing your coffee, always go with organic—coffee is one of the most heavily sprayed crops.

2. **EGCG.** Epigallocatechin gallate is a polyphenol found in green tea that works synergistically with caffeine to increase heat production in the body and to amplify the effect of the catecholamines. Therapeutic levels are 270 milligrams of EGCG per day, which is beyond what could be consumed by drinking green tea, no matter how cold it is outside. Supplementation is your best option here.

3. **CLA.** Conjugated linoleic acid is a naturally occurring derivative of linoleic acid, an omega-6 essential fatty acid (but it does not add omega-6 to the diet, which is a good thing). CLA has been shown to increase metabolic rate, reduce insulin, and improve glucose tolerance, all essential components to losing fat from around the

midsection. A therapeutic amount is 3400 milligrams per day in divided doses.

4. **L-carnatine.** L-carnatine is used to aid in the transport of fat to muscle cells, where it can then be used for energy production. This results in increased performance as well as improvements in fat loss. L-carnatine is best taken with fish oil or starch-based carbs like potato or rice. The recommended dosage is 2 to 4 grams daily.

5. **Alpha lipoic acid (ALA).** This potent antioxidant has been shown to increase energy, performance, and metabolism. Look for the "R" form (not the "S" form), and use it in conjunction with L-carnatine.

6. **Yohimbe.** Often touted as being a male sexual performance supplement, yohimbe is actually great for both sexes, since it increases blood flow (as opposed to increasing testosterone, as was once believed). Yohimbe works to inhibit the alpha receptors, allowing for the catecholamines to do their job of releasing stored fat more effectively. If you recall, the only other way to inhibit your alpha receptors is by consuming a low-carb diet. Yohimbe can be used to amplify the effect of eating fewer carbs, *or* you can try using it in conjunction with a regular, balanced diet. Caution must be used when using this supplement, as it is a stimulant and will increase heart rate and feelings of anxiety. When used in conjunction with a low-carb diet and exercise, yohimbe can certainly aid in the release of fat from your trouble spots. Studies have shown effective results using 10 milligrams twice daily for three weeks. Other experts recommend a more precise dose of 0.44 milligrams per pound of body weight. If you want to try yohimbe, look for the standardized HCl version and start with a very

low dose, taken about a half hour before exercise and at least three hours after a meal.

7. **Coleus forskohlii.** This tropical perennial plant activates an enzyme that increases the hormone cAMP and, as you may recall, cAMP plays an important role in the release of trouble spot fat from cells. Coleus forskohlii also normalizes thyroid hormone production while stimulating its release. One of the great things about Coleus forskohlii is that it does not stimulate the central nervous system like other thermogenics, such as ephedrine, so it is well tolerated and safe to use. Use in conjunction with hydroxycitric acid (HCA) and ALA for maximum benefit.

8. **Ephedrine.** I mentioned this popular over-the-counter stimulant at the beginning of the chapter. This beta agonist stimulates beta receptors and causes the body to release adrenaline, which increases temperature, heart rate, and the release of free fatty acids into the bloodstream. Some experts claim that it also has anticatabolic effects. Ephedrine works very well but only for a short period. With prolonged use, receptors will downgrade, reducing its effectiveness. I am not a big fan of using ephedrine simply because the side effects are a bit too much for me. There have been some deaths associated with its use, so if you choose to use it, exercise caution and never use it in conjunction with yohimbe.

9. **Hydroxycitric acid (HCA).** This is found in several tropical plants, including Garcinia cambogia. HCA helps reduce appetite, inhibits the conversion of carbohydrates (sugars) into fat, and improves the rate of fat burning in cells by inhibiting an enzyme that blocks fat from being burned. I use a formulation that contains

HCA, Coleus forskohlii, ALA, and caffeine twice daily during a fat-loss phase.

10. **Calcium.** Research shows that supplemental calcium can aid in fat loss with the added bonus of increasing testosterone levels. If you are deficient, try supplementing with 500 milligrams per day.

SUPPLEMENTS FOR ENHANCED MUSCLE GAINS

As you will soon discover, building muscle mass is actually more fun than losing body fat. This is because building muscle requires a calorie surplus—a fancy way of saying that you get to eat more healthy food (especially carbs). With more healthy food comes more nutrients, and more nutrients means that there is a reduced need for supplements. Some programs may require you to purchase the latest, greatest muscle-building potion, but the truth is that nothing is more anabolic than food, training, and rest. Not even a supplement (with the exception of anabolic steroids). That being said, there are two supplements you may want to consider adding to those in the Tier 1 list.

1. **A good-quality multivitamin/multimineral.** When you are working on creating new tissue, it may be useful to enlist the help of some additional nutrients. I use a multivitamin/multimineral in the morning on my heavy training days.

2. **Creatine.** Creatine supplement has been around for more than a decade. When I first used it, I was surprised by how well it worked to increase my lean body mass. I was never able to repeat those same results with subsequent use. However, many studies support its effectiveness in increasing strength and performance. New research also suggests that

creatine supplementation may be useful for preventing depression, neurological disease, memory loss, and even diabetes. At one time, creatine was expensive, but now it is dirt cheap by comparison. It is safe and well tolerated by most people (provided they stick to the recommended dose; those with kidney disease should consult their physician before using it). I should also caution that too much creatine can produce unpredictable and explosive results in the bathroom, so don't say I didn't warn you. That being said, 5 grams daily is generally well tolerated and what is usually prescribed.

SUPPLEMENTS FOR ENHANCED PERFORMANCE

Increasing performance is something every athlete or weekend warrior is interested in accomplishing. Performance can be measured in many ways, including speed, distance, strength, endurance, and mobility. Improvements in sport performance can carry over to everyday activities. Below I've listed some supplements that have been proven to help. For improved performance, add these to your Tier 1 list.

1. **L-carnatine.** This is one of those supplements you have to experiment with to see if it works for you. Some people swear by it and claim it improves cognitive functioning and increases motivation to train. One thing that L-carnatine can help with for sure is removing lactic acid, which builds up during intense training and can definitively limit performance. L-carnatine helps reduce this buildup while also decreasing inflammation, making it a good supplement to try if you are interested in increasing endurance. It is best taken with fish oil or starch-based carbs like potato or rice. The recommended dosage is 2 to 4 grams daily.

2. **Digestive enzymes.** There are three types of enzymes: systemic enzymes (which are produced by the body and necessary for life), digestive enzymes, and food enzymes (which must be obtained from the foods we eat). Food energy is required to fuel activity; however, food must be digested to make the energy-providing nutrients available. If digestion is poor, foods will not be properly broken down, and your body will not obtain the nutrients it needs. Digestion of food relies on enzymes, and a deficiency of enzymes leads to poor digestion. Taking digestive enzymes improves the rate at which nutrients are broken down, allowing for their faster absorption and use by working muscles. Our body's natural production of enzymes decreases with age and, combined with cooking food (which destroys enzymes), this makes supplementation necessary. I recommend taking enzymes at the beginning of each meal.

3. **Antioxidants.** Antioxidants such as vitamin E, selenium, zinc, beta carotene, and vitamin C are needed to reduce inflammation and oxidative stress. Oxidative stress happens when the body produces free radicals in response to the oxygen-rich environment formed by increased respiration. These free radicals must be neutralized before they go on to damage cells, which can lead to inflammation and accelerated aging. Increased amounts of aerobic exercise can cause chronic inflammation, thus necessitating the use of supplemental antioxidants. Fruits such as raspberries, strawberries, and cherries have also been shown to have anti-inflammatory effects in athletes.

4. **Beta-alanine.** This amino acid has been shown to boost exercise performance. The supplement helps clear fatiguing hydrogen ions that are produced with

high-intensity exercise. According to research, beta-alanine has demonstrated improvements in performance during multiple bouts of high-intensity exercise and in single bouts of exercise lasting more than 60 seconds. These results suggest that beta-alanine may increase your anaerobic threshold and time to exhaustion—so it's definitely worth a try if your goal is to improve performance. The ideal dosage is 4 grams per day.

5. **Activfuel+.** This drink is a blend of performance-enhancing ingredients to be used immediately before and during exercise. Activfuel+ contains organic red beet juice, which dilates blood vessels and increases oxygen delivery to cells. One study showed an increase in endurance of 16% using beet juice alone. Activfuel+ also contains BCAAs, coconut water (high in electrolytes), caffeine (for increased performance and focus), creatine, and B vitamins. I have used this product extensively and find it to be excellent for increasing muscular endurance. For a somewhat similar effect you could also use a combination of concentrated beet juice powder, creatine, and caffeine along with your vitamin supplements.

SUPPLEMENTS FOR REDUCING PAIN

Anybody who has been training consistently for a year or two will likely be able to remember experiencing minor acute injuries from time to time. Several vitamin and mineral supplements, as well as a topical cream, can help with acute-injury recovery.

1. **A good-quality multivitamin/multimineral.** Take twice per day (morning and evening) to provide your body with the vitamins and minerals needed in the healing process.

2. **Fish oil.** If you are already following my Tier 1 recommendations or otherwise taking up to 6 grams of fish oil a day, you will not need to increase your dosage, but if you are not already taking fish oil as a supplement, use 6 to 10 grams daily to help reduce inflammation. Omega-6 oils should be kept to a minimum, though, as they are pro-inflammatory.

3. **Curcumin.** This is the active ingredient found in turmeric, a plant well known for its healing properties. The simplest way to include curcumin in your diet is to take supplemental turmeric extract three times per day.

4. **Traumeel.** This is a homeopathic preparation used to relieve muscular and joint pain, inflammation, and bruising associated with injuries.

5. **Natural eggshell membrane (NEM).** Try this supplement if you are experiencing joint or muscle pain. NEM is the white film you find around a hard-boiled egg when you peel it. Researchers discovered that this stuff is rich in chemicals that aid in pain reduction while also helping rebuild cartilage in the joints. The bonus is that there are no side effects or contraindications to using NEM, so it is safe for all to use. I recommend a product called fast back care+. In addition to NEM, fast back care+ contains white willow and devil's claw for additional pain relief.

6. **Proteolytic enzymes.** Enzymes can help with more than just your digestion. They can also speed up healing. The proteolytic enzymes papain and bromelain (found in papaya and pineapples) are natural anti-inflammatories and have been shown to reduce pain, increase blood flow, and "digest" damaged tissue that accumulates as a result of an injury.

PART FOUR
YOUR BODY PLUS THE MUSCLE

10

Carb Feasting

The Fastest Way to Gain 10 Pounds of Muscle

It was March 6, 2009, when I got the call. On the phone was Craig Charity, editor of *Revive* magazine. He had some good news for me. Craig was looking for a male fitness expert for the cover of his summer issue and wondered if I was interested. Needless to say, I was honored. But I had a problem. I was going through a very difficult period in my life during which I experienced a lot of personal disappointment and, because of a legal dispute, saw my income disappear. The stress was taking its toll, and I found myself losing weight at an alarming rate. In less than five months, I had dropped nearly 20 pounds of lean mass. My health deteriorated quickly, and I was suffering from internal and external bleeding (I'll spare you the gory details) and expressing symptoms similar to an aggressive form of cancer.

For the first time in my life, I was scared about my health. I spent several months visiting various doctors and specialists. One of the great things about Canada is that you don't pay out of pocket for a doctor-ordered MRI. One of the crappy things is that you may have to wait months for an appointment.

The tests came back negative for cancer but positive for stress. It is simply amazing how stress can manifest itself in the body. Armed with a powerful sense of relief that I wasn't terminally ill and newfound conviction, I shifted my attention away from the problems I was experiencing and began implementing many of the techniques discussed in this book. I focused on getting my body back into shape physically and emotionally, and in doing so was able to show up on the day of the photo shoot in better shape than before all the shit hit the fan in my life.

Here is a picture from the day of that shoot:

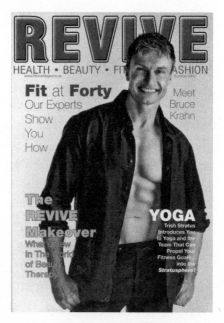

On this day I weighed 200 pounds
and was 8% body fat.

One of the things I found interesting while I experienced those symptoms I told you about was how quickly body composition can change. During my slump, in a very short period of time I managed to not only lose almost 20 pounds of muscle but also gain approximately 5 pounds of fat. The opportunity for a magazine cover was very motivating for me, and reversing the damage to my body in as little time as possible became my new goal. In this chapter I am going to explain to you exactly how I did it.

NEW-SCHOOL MUSCLE GAIN

Gaining muscle without gaining fat is the goal of any athlete. Muscle means strength and speed, whereas fat means excess weight and decreased performance. The old-school method of bulking up by gaining pounds of excess fat along with some muscle is an antiquated approach. This is the new world of muscle building—muscle building 2.0—and it allows for more lean muscle without the extra fat. Welcome to body composition utopia.

YOUNG AND DUMB

There is a lot of talk about losing body fat but very little about building muscle. The fact is that most people grossly undervalue the importance of increasing lean body mass—young, impressionable males making the biggest exception to this rule. I can recall the first time I saw a picture of Arnold Schwarzenegger. I was 13 years old and watched the movie *Pumping Iron* for the first time. Arnold appeared larger than life and seemed to epitomize everything a young man could ever want out of life—strength, confidence, influence, fame, and fortune. And at the very heart of his seemingly endless ambitions and abilities were his *muscles*.

I began my pursuit of muscle mass relatively young in an attempt to free myself from a battle with low self-esteem, negativity, and cursed muscle-building genetics. I'm not from the best stock when it comes to athleticism. When I look at my relatives, not one could be described as athletic. A more appropriate description would be "slim" (a nice word for "skinny"). My lack of muscle and seemingly inadequate ability to gain lean mass is painfully obvious when you compare me with the average male. According to statistics (and the observations of numerous strength coaches), with proper training, the average male will put on anywhere from 1 to 2 pounds of muscle per month (12 to 24 pounds total) in the first year of training.

How much did I gain in my first year of training?

Nothing. I actually *lost* weight.

That's right. Despite working out diligently and taking copious amounts of dubious supplements, I managed to gain nothing. Nada. Zilch. El zippo.

Looking back now, I am not surprised. At the time, I was following the training programs outlined in various muscle magazines, as well as those found in every male teenager's bodybuilding bible, *Encyclopedia of Modern Bodybuilding*, by Arnold Schwarzenegger. Although the programs outlined in those publications may work for athletes who are, shall we say, *chemically enhanced*, they will do little for average joes who are taking nothing beyond creatine and protein powder.

HOW MUCH MUSCLE CAN *YOU* GAIN?

Several factors are involved in determining how much muscle you can build and at what rate:

1. **How long have you been training?**
   This is the single most important factor. A 30-year-old who has been training consistently and intelligently for 10 years will have far less muscle-building potential than a 30-year-old who has never lifted before. I say "intelligently" because if your lifting program consists of nothing more than planks, push-ups, and Bosu ball training, you are probably nowhere near your genetic limit. During the past two decades of training clients, I have

discovered that there is an inverse relationship between training age and the amount of muscle one can build.

YEARS OF CONSISTENT, INTELLIGENT TRAINING	POTENTIAL AMOUNT OF MUSCLE
1	2 pounds per month
2	1 pound per month
3	6 pounds per year
4	2 to 3 pounds per year
5+	Reached genetic limit

Note: These numbers represent the average male. Female potential for muscle gain will be approximately half.

2. **What are your testosterone levels?**
   Testosterone is your body's key muscle-building hormone, and levels fluctuate widely from person to person. According to research, men aren't what they used to be, as testosterone levels in males are dropping by an average of 1.2% per year. That is a staggering decrease and will have a profound effect on body composition. A hormone-boosting training program and intelligent diet will help optimize your levels, but in many cases, further intervention is necessary. The only way to know where you stand is to have your hormone levels analyzed using a simple blood test. Ask your doctor to arrange for testing. I have had clients in their 20s who tested very low for their age.

3. **Who are your parents?**
   Genetics play a large role in your muscle-building potential. Some men can build muscle by just looking at the weights, whereas others struggle to have arms that resemble something other than toothpicks. Most of us are average and fall somewhere in between these two extremes. Nothing you can do here except blame your parents I guess . . .

4. **What is your training history?**
   I have helped many people complete body transformations. The ones who have the "easiest" transformation are those who were in great shape, let themselves go, and then got back into great shape. I know from experience that I have little problem regaining any muscle I may lose because of illness or inactivity. This is because of muscle memory. Breaking new ground is an entirely different story.

MUSCLE-BUILDING MISTAKES

If there is one thing I am known for, it's persistence. When I set my heart and mind on something, I simply do not quit until I attain it. Fortunately for me, when it came to building muscle, this was the sole reason for my eventual success. Despite my rocky start, I finally figured out what works and what doesn't and in the process gained more than 40 pounds of solid muscle. But before I tell you what works, I want to identify the most common mistakes men and women make when trying to increase lean muscle mass.

Chasing Two Rabbits

At first, I wanted to look like the guys in the magazines, all of whom had big, ripped muscles. In other words, I wanted to get bigger and lose fat. The problem with this approach is that gaining muscle and losing fat are conflicting goals: gaining muscle requires a calorie surplus, and losing fat requires a calorie deficit. This is what I mean by "chasing two rabbits." The look I was shooting for simply wasn't possible given my lack of muscle. I needed to focus on building up a solid foundation of muscle first and then change my approach to one of fat loss. I'm a bit of an unusual case, though. Most people need to lose fat first before they will experience the real benefits of muscle building. But when it is time to build, the fear of gaining even an ounce of fat is what holds back many men and women whose goal is to have more muscle. I want you to put that fear behind you during this phase of the program. By now you should have significantly reduced your body fat stores and your body is primed to gain muscle. And you can always go back to the fat-loss program if you find you need to after the muscle-building phase.

Not Eating Enough Food

Show me a person who says they can't gain muscular body weight and I will show you someone who probably isn't eating enough. Gaining body weight is a mathematical certainty if sufficient calories are consumed. Of course, we are not looking to gain pounds of flab—it's lean muscle we are after, and that's where the correct training program comes in. When I embarked on my journey to regain the weight I had lost because of my illness, I had to break down some mental barriers that stood in my mind surrounding food. Up until that time, I ate small meals frequently throughout the day. Many years of doing so had programmed my body to develop a metabolic set point regarding meal patterns and calories consumed. I was accustomed to eating small portions and was unable to consume large meals without feeling sick. I remedied this by simply increasing the amount of food I ate in my post-exercise meal a little each time. Often, I would accelerate the process by *drinking* more calories in the same period as well. Simple, effective, and oh so enjoyable!

SIMPLE POST-WORKOUT MUSCLE-GAIN SHAKE

This baby is high in quality protein, fiber, and good fats, all in a tasty formula. Drinking one of these after each workout will provide your body with lots of calories, and kick-start the muscle-building process. All you need is a blender and a few basic ingredients.

3 to 5 ice cubes

½ cup frozen fruit

2 scoops protein powder (or 1 scoop protein powder and ½ cup cottage cheese if you like a very thick shake)

1 serving greens+ or other green food supplement

⅓ cup mixed raw nuts

5 grams creatine

1 cup unsweetened coconut, almond, or hemp milk

Following Too Many "Gurus"

As great as the Internet is as a source of information, so much of what's on it can actually work against you. There are millions of pages of muscle-building info online, and the surplus can lead to paralysis by analysis. Sometimes it's better to forget everything you may have believed to be true and simply start moving forward with a plan. For the next four weeks, step away from the magazines, websites, forums, and books (except this one, of course!) and commit yourself to this program 100%. You will be amazed by how great it feels to liberate your mind from the doubt and confusion once and for all.

Too Much High-Intensity Cardio

Have you ever seen a muscular marathon runner? The answer is no, and here's why: excessive cardio is a surefire recipe for muscle loss. The entire Trouble Spot Fat Loss program is built on the fact that your body can only adapt maximally in one direction at a time. During a muscle-building phase, the focus should be more on activities that produce tissue growth (resistance training) and less on activities that promote tissue breakdown (cardio).

Even playing sports too often can sidetrack your muscle-growth goals. Muscles typically need 48 hours of rest to adapt to the stresses placed on them during intense training. Engaging in too many extracurricular cardio activities makes your body more likely to use any excess calories it has for fuel and not for building new tissue.

Limit cardiovascular activity to 20 minutes of low-intensity work, three times a week *max*, during this phase. In fact, it is best to start with no cardio and see what effect that has on your body. If you find yourself gaining fat, you can always include 20 minutes after one of your resistance-training workouts.

Not Measuring Progress the Correct Way

Remember, whatever gets measured gets managed. These are the four measurements you need to monitor while in a muscle-gaining phase:

1. **How much weight you are lifting.** Muscle gains follow strength, but the reverse is not always true. I want you to focus during this phase of the program on increasing the weights you lift at each workout. Even small incremental increases in weight lifted will prove to be beneficial.

2. **How many meals you are eating.** To increase muscle size, your body requires an increase in calories consumed. I have always had a difficult time consuming large amounts of food at one sitting and find it much easier to simply eat an extra meal or two each day. During a fat-loss phase, eating two to three times per day can work well, but when trying to increase muscle, a higher meal frequency is often better.

3. **How much you weigh.** In this phase, you will need to see the reading on the scale move up each week. Immediately following a fat-loss phase, your body is primed to grow lean tissue, so the scale reading should be moving up, not down. If you are not gaining weight, simply increase your portions and/or meal frequency until you see your weight start to move.

4. **How big your waist is.** During this phase, you want to make sure that the increases in body weight are mostly muscle with minimal fat. The easiest way to track this (without performing an actual body composition analysis) is by monitoring your waist measurement. If you are gaining weight too fast and notice that your waist circumference has increased by more than an inch

or two, take a moment to reevaluate your eating habits. Some fat gain is acceptable (just like some muscle loss is inevitable when training for maximum fat loss), but this must be kept to a minimum. If your waist suddenly balloons up from 32 inches to 35 inches, it's an indication that your calorie intake is too high.

Training by Gender Instead of Goals

Men and women have more similarities than differences, and yet for some reason, women are often told that they should train differently from a man who shares the same goal. The media perpetuates this myth by telling women that some forms of exercise are best for toning while others are best for bulking. This is complete nonsense and along the same lines as the claims made by certain programs that they will lengthen existing muscles or create long and lean ones. A basic physiology book will quickly show you that the places where a given muscle attaches to the bone (the origin and insertion) are fixed and cannot be changed. Yoga is a great complement to a resistance-training program, but some of the claims surrounding its fat-loss and muscle-building benefits are a tad bit off. What I am saying is that, regardless of whether you're male or female, the exercises to be done are the same. What may be different are the exercise protocols, but those are dependent on the goal you want to achieve, not on your gender. (See "Train by Your Goal, Not by Your Gender" in chapter 8 for further discussion of this.)

Training Only the Muscles You Love

According to strength-training coach (and my brother) Bryan Krahn, CSCS, one of the most common mistakes he observes new trainees (and even some seasoned gym veterans) making is training only the muscles they see in the mirror, namely the shoulders, arms, chest (if a guy)—and, of course, the abs. Although everyone wants to develop these muscles—and they're certainly fun to train—exercising just the "showy" body parts leaves the biggest muscle groups out of the equation, typically the legs and back. These muscles burn a ton of calories, and when developed, greatly improve the visual appeal of your physique. (Think about it: Is there anything sillier than seeing someone with a big, muscular upper body and pencil-thin legs?) Aesthetics aside, there's also your health to consider, namely something called structural balance. Your body performs best when the entire musculature is developed and strong, and ignoring this can result in serious issues. For example, if you train your shoulders and chest and forget about the opposing muscles (the posterior deltoids and upper back), your posture can suffer considerably. The result can be the dreaded forward-protruding-head look, which is great if you aspire to resemble a Neanderthal scanning the pavement for loose change. Bottom line: exercise the whole body, not just the parts that look good in the mirror.

HOW TO INCREASE CALORIES FOR MORE MUSCLE WITHOUT GETTING FAT

I cannot tell you how many times I have heard a skinny guy or gal tell me that they cannot gain weight. If your training program is even somewhat intelligent, the most likely reason for your lack of muscle-building progress is *insufficient calorie intake*. The good news is that fixing this is not only easy, it can be pleasurable too.

Eating for more muscle growth involves making two small but critical changes to your fat-loss diet:

1. You must increase your calories.
2. You must increase your carbohydrate intake.

Instead of going hog wild and slurping down loads of pasta at each meal, I prefer to take a more systematic approach. By doing so, I can control how fast I gain weight, and this helps ensure that the extra pounds I add are primarily muscle, with the least amount of fat. In the past, bodybuilders were known to follow extreme "bulk and cut" cycles, and it was not uncommon to see some of them approaching obesity during the off season.

This is not an option for me, nor should it be for you. The goal here is to gain quality lean muscle mass, not slabs of fat that you will have to starve off later. It is perfectly acceptable to have collateral damage in the form of some body fat gain during this phase, but if you do it the way I am describing, nobody will notice the fat—they will just notice how awesome you look.

The eating guidelines below are not that different from those you learned about in chapter 7. The most significant change is in the frequency and amount of carbohydrates you will be eating. The trick to increasing carbs and calories without increasing body fat is to eat them at the correct time. If you simply ate more oatmeal, rice, and potatoes with each meal of the day, you would likely gain weight, most of it in the form of body fat. However, if you time it so that you consume those foods *only* in the *post*-exercise period, your body will partition more of those nutrients toward muscle building and repair instead of to your love handles. By saving the majority of your calories and carbs for after your workout, you will be taking advantage of the hormone insulin as well as of the glucose transporter GLUT4, both of which can shuttle nutrients preferentially toward muscle cells instead of toward fat cells.

Making this work for you is easier than it sounds. Here are the rules you need to follow:

1. Start your day with a breakfast consisting of black coffee (or green tea), a palm-sized portion of raw nuts

(e.g., Brazil, almond, or walnuts; or you could have 5 to 10 grams of fish oil if you prefer), and 20 to 40 grams of protein (whole food is best, but BCAAs or whey/vegetarian-based protein will work too). It's a good idea to cycle your protein sources, so feel free to vary the nuts and type of protein you choose daily. This breakfast is excellent for increasing fat burning and mental focus. The typical North American breakfast consisting of juices and grain products does the exact opposite.

2. Each of your pre-workout meals should consist primarily of protein, fats, and green vegetables. Keep fruits to a bare minimum too. As for meal frequency, it's up to you. I prefer a meal frequency higher than when in a fat-loss phase for two reasons:

   • Eating more often makes it easier to consume more calories for building muscle.

   • The increase in meal frequency allows for more frequent insulin spikes. Insulin may temporarily impede fat burning, but it is also an anabolic hormone and potent muscle builder.

3. Pre-workout, consume 5 to 10 grams of BCAAs and, optionally, 50 to 150 milligrams of caffeine. If possible, schedule your workouts for late afternoon or early evening, as strength tends to be greatest during this period (plus this leaves time for you to have a post-workout feast).

4. During your workout, sip on water mixed with BCAAs. This will help keep you energized while preventing muscle catabolism.

5. Post-workout, consume your post-workout muscle-gain shake (see page 185).

6. About an hour after your post-workout drink, consume a meal high in protein *and* carbohydrates and *low* in fat.

My preference is for these carbs to be quick-digesting—for example, white potato or white rice—and to contain very little fat. This is also a good time to include any foods you may be craving, but don't turn each post-workout meal into a free-for-all. The rate at which you gain body fat will determine how liberal you can be with your food selections.

7. Because you are working on building muscle, it is important that you increase calories. Therefore, from the first meal an hour after you work out until you go to bed, continue to consume meals that combine lean protein and carbohydrates with minimal amounts of fat.

8. For those of you who want to crunch the numbers, your target calorie intake during a muscle-building phase is approximately your body weight × 15 kcal per day. This is where you should start, but the number may have to be increased depending on how your body responds.

Muscle-Building Calorie Guide

BODY WEIGHT	DAILY CALORIE INTAKE (-/+ 10% RANGE)
100 lb	1500 kcal (1350–1650 kcal)
150 lb	2250 kcal (2025–2475 kcal)
200 lb	3000 kcal (2700–3300 kcal)
250 lb	3750 kcal (3375–4125 kcal)
300 lb	4500 kcal (4050–4950 kcal)

If you find that the weight isn't coming on fast enough, simply increase the portion sizes of your post-workout meals (see general portion guidelines below). Do the opposite if you are gaining excessive amounts of body fat, but remember, some body fat gain during a muscle-building phase is acceptable.

PORTION GUIDELINES DURING A MUSCLE-BUILDING PHASE

Women: Each pre-workout meal should consist of:
- 1 palm-sized portion of protein
- 1 fist-sized portion of vegetables
- 1 thumb-sized portion of fats

Men: Each pre-workout meal should consist of:
- 2 palm-sized portions of protein
- 2 fist-sized portions of vegetables
- 2 thumb-sized portions of fats

Women: Each post-workout meal should consist of:
- 1 palm-sized portion of protein
- 1 fist-sized portion of vegetables
- 1 palm-sized portion of healthy carbs

Men: Each post-workout meal should consist of:
- 2 palm-sized portions of protein
- 2 fist-sized portions of vegetables
- 2 palm-sized portions of healthy carbs

Note: The number of carbohydrate-rich meals you should consume during the post-workout period depends on two variables: the time of day that you exercise and your carbohydrate tolerance. For example, if you are a person who trains at six o'clock in the morning, you may have your first post-workout, carbohydrate-rich, whole food meal at eight o'clock. But what about the rest of the day's meals? Should they all be high in carbs as well? The answer is generally not. It does depend on the individual, but I have found that typically the best approach is to include starch-based carbs with the first *two* meals after your workout, and then switch back to consuming proteins, veggies, and healthy fats only. Some people, however, have excellent carbohydrate sensitivity and can tolerate a greater number of carbohydrate-rich meals. The only way to know for sure is to experiment with different serving frequencies and track your results. Although, for an individual who is very carb sensitive and prefers to exercise in the morning, it still may be preferable to have only one high-carb meal per day. In this case, save it for the evening, to allow for better overall insulin management. And, of course, if you're working out in the late afternoon or evening, you may have only one post-workout meal anyway.

For those who prefer a more scientific answer to the carbohydrate question, I give you this: research suggests that the ideal amount of carbohydrates needed for replenishing muscle glycogen (without excess fat gain) is 1.76 grams of carbs per 1 pound of body weight.

CYCLE YOUR CALORIES TO PREVENT FAT GAIN

Important: When training to gain muscle, follow the high-calorie eating phase for a maximum of four weeks. At the end of this period, revert back to the carb-fasting program and reduce your calorie and carbohydrate intake for one week before returning to your higher-calorie, carb-feasting program. Interjecting timed weeks of reduced carbohydrates and calories will help your body maintain insulin sensitivity and serve to keep your body fat levels to a minimum while in a muscle-building phase.

TRAINING FOR MUSCLE GROWTH

There are two types of muscle growth, or hypertrophy, as it is also known: *sarcoplasmic* and *myofibrillar.*

Sarcoplasmic hypertrophy is the increase in the volume of noncontractile protein and fluid between muscle fibers. This is the type of "growth" that occurs with lightweight, high-rep training. In bodybuilding terms, it's known as "the pump." The buildup of fluid causes a temporary increase in muscle size that lasts for up to an hour or two and causes the muscles to look bigger. This is why Saturdays are always chest and back day at the gym, as guys "pump up" before heading out to the bar wearing a shirt they bought at Gap Kids . . . but I digress.

Myofibrillar hypertrophy is more functional than sarcoplasmic, involving as it does an increase in the actual number of muscle fibers (density) and an increase in contractile protein. This type of muscle growth better indicates strength and is more permanent (if the training remains consistent). Myofibrillar hypertrophy occurs when training is performed using heavier loads, low reps (approximately 6 or fewer), and lots of sets.

For muscle growth, it is important to vary rep ranges in order to stimulate the full gamut of muscle fibers. Varying rep ranges is also best for anabolic hormone release, stimulating an increase in testosterone, growth hormone, and *insulin-like growth factor-1*, a substance the body produces that promotes muscle growth. If you rely on training methods that use only a single rep range, you will not experience maximal muscle growth because you won't recruit all the available muscle fibers.

In addition to rep range, there are several other factors to consider when training for muscle growth, discussed below.

Sets

There is an inverse relationship between sets and reps. The higher the number of repetitions, the fewer the number of sets that should be performed. Lately, there has been a resurgence of the old "one set to failure" protocol for maximum muscle gains. Proponents of this system believe that a single set of maximal effort is all that is required to stimulate growth. Sounds great, but this method tends to work only for beginners with little training experience. For people with more than two months' training under their belts, more sets are required to bring about growth. Use the following guidelines to determine how many sets you should be doing:

LENGTH OF REGULAR TRAINING	NUMBER OF SETS PER EXERCISE
Less than 2 months	1–2
2 to 6 months	2–4
6 months or more	4–6

Tempo

As you know from chapter 8, tempo is the speed of each repetition. What you may not know is that tempo is possibly the single most overlooked training variable. Overlooking tempo is a shame, since small manipulations to tempo can bring about big results. Throwing the weights around all willy-nilly, with no regard for the speed at which you raise or lower them, is not the right way to do things. Tempo is so important that it dictates the weights you use and the number of reps you must hit. With the *Trouble Spot Fat Loss* muscle-building workouts, every single working set should be *very, very hard* to finish. This will help keep the workouts short and effective.

As I explain in chapter 8, tempo is often illustrated using a sequence of three digits. The first digit refers to the lowering (negative) movement, the middle digit refers to the pause (sometimes denoted as "0," meaning no pause), and the third digit refers to the return (positive) movement. "X" is used to denote "as fast as possible." For example, "2-1-2" indicates lowering the weight in 2 seconds, pausing at the bottom 1 second, and raising the weight in 2 seconds. Tempo can and should be varied, even within the same workout. Follow the tempo guidelines for the workouts described below.

TEMPO GUIDELINES	
First exercise	4-0-X
Second exercise	3-0-X
Third exercise	2-0-X

Rest Interval

The amount of time you spend resting between each exercise and set of exercises is crucial to getting the most of the workout. The goal is to keep the rest intervals relatively brief by resting only 10 seconds between exercises and 2 minutes between each set. There is no need for long, drawn-out workouts. We are going to keep the workouts brief and intense by packing lots of work into a relatively short period. With this workout, you will perform three exercises in a row (referred to as a "circuit"), resting only 10 seconds between each exercise. The exercises within each circuit are listed as A1, A2, and A3. Repeat each circuit for the recommended number of sets given your length of regular training, as shown in the chart on page 196.

Exercise Selection

Choosing the correct exercises for building muscle is actually simple. As with the exercises for fat loss, five primary movements will make up the majority of your exercise program: squatting, pushing, pulling, lunging, and total body. Secondary exercises for the elbow flexors and extensors, as well as lateral raises and abdominal movements, are also included. A quick search on YouTube will reveal thousands of exercises within these categories. Below, I present you with the exercises that I feel produce the greatest results, but by no means is this selection meant to be final. You will likely have to make adjustments according to what equipment is available to you.

Frequency

With this program you will train 4 days out of 7. You can structure your workouts in one of several ways. Generally, I never like to train with weights more than 3 days in a row without having a rest day to allow for recovery. Even though we will be working specific areas of the body to allow for greater volume and intensity for each body part, the intense nature of this program necessitates adequate rest and recovery. Here is an overview of how often you will be training in a week.

Day 1: Workout

Day 2: Workout

Day 3: Off

Day 4: Workout

Day 5: Off

Day 6: Workout

Day 7: Off

Repeat for a *maximum* of 6 to 8 weeks, after which, return to the fat loss phase if needed, or start the maintenance phase desribed in chapter 12.

Change Your Focus

During this phase, you will concentrate on building more muscle, and this requires a different mental focus. When training for sarcoplasmic and myofibrillar hypertrophy, it is important to feel the muscle being worked, not the weight you're lifting. At first, this may sound silly, but to brush off this instruction would be a mistake. The better able you are to actually feel the muscle you are training, the faster that muscle will develop.

The key to accomplishing this is to shift your focus from the external (the weight) to the internal (the muscles). For example, for bicep curls, focus your mind on the inside of your elbow flexors. Focus on the force of the contraction as you curl the dumbbell, and the stretch as you lower it. Flex your antagonistic muscles (in this case, the triceps) as you hit the bottom position. Use this technique through each exercise and you will see what a difference it can make.

THE 6-12-25 PROTOCOL FOR MUSCLE GROWTH

This is by far the hardest muscle-building workout I have ever completed. The method was first introduced to the bodybuilding world by Charles Poliquin, who is a master at manipulating the human body for increased size and strength. As they say, the devil is in the details, and so it is with this simple yet oh-so-effective program. With this workout you will be hitting your muscles from various positions of flexion and tempos, and through a broad spectrum of rep ranges. Feel free to swap out exercises as necessary, but try sticking closely to the theme outlined below. The major benefit of the 6-12-25 Protocol is that it incorporates a variety of loads—increasing strength, muscularity, and endurance all in one workout. Be prepared to feel the burn, literally. This workout produces lots of lactic acid, which has a positive effect on growth hormone levels as well as on aerobic capacity. You will also experience a tremendous "pump" of blood rushing to your working muscles as a combination of growth hormone, cellular swelling, and muscle damage creates the ideal environment for muscle growth. In this workout you will perform 6 reps for strength, 12 reps for muscular growth, and then finish with 25 reps for muscular endurance. The key to making this work properly is selecting the correct weights for each of the exercises: heavy weight for the first set of 6 reps, moderate weight for the second set of 12 reps, and lighter weight for the final set of 25 reps. At the end of each set, you should be at or very near your maximum limit. If you feel that you could squeeze out an extra 2 or 3 reps, the weight is too light, and if you fall short of the goal reps by 1 or 2, the weight is too heavy. As you progress and become stronger you will need to increase the amount of weight in your lifts. This is a good thing, since increased muscle size almost always follows an increase in strength.

NOTE:

- The order in which each body part is trained in the daily workouts outlined below is not set in stone. I always suggest beginning with your weakest body part first. For example, if you are training triceps and biceps, and your biceps are lagging in development, begin the workout by training your biceps first.

- Between each exercise in each circuit (e.g., between A1, A2, and A3), rest for 10 seconds, and rest for two minutes before repeating the circuit.

- Repeat the circuit one to five times, depending on your training experience (see page 196).

WARM-UP CIRCUIT

- Begin with a 3-to-5-minute cardio warm-up of your choice (biking, running, skipping, etc.).
- Next, complete 2 rounds of the following:
  - Lying hip extension × 15 reps
  - Bird dog × 10 per side
  - Y squat × 10

6-12-25 PROTOCOL FOR MUSCLE BUILDING

Workout 1

	SHOULDERS AND ABS	# REPS	TEMPO
A1	Standing shoulder press with barbell	6	4-0-X
A2	Seated dumbbell Arnold press	12	3-0-X
A3	Seated lateral raise	25	2-0-X
	REST 2 MINUTES. REPEAT 1 TO 5 MORE TIMES		
B1	Reverse crunch	6	4-0-X
B2	Incline crunch on stability ball	12	3-0-X
B3	Abdominal knee tuck on stability ball	25	2-0-X
	REST 2 MINUTES. REPEAT 1 TO 5 MORE TIMES		

Workout 2

	TRICEPS AND BICEPS	# REPS	TEMPO
A1	Triceps dip	6	4-0-X
A2	Lying triceps extension with dumbbells	12	3-0-X
A3	Seated overhead dumbbell extension	25	2-0-X
	REST 2 MINUTES. REPEAT 1 TO 5 MORE TIMES		
B1	Standing bicep curl (reverse grip using an EZ curl bar)	6	4-0-X
B2	Incline dumbbell hammer curl	12	3-0-X
B3	Preacher curl with stability ball	25	2-0-X
	REST 2 MINUTES. REPEAT 1 TO 5 MORE TIMES		

Workout 3

	LOWER BODY	# REPS	TEMPO
A1	Barbell squat	6	4-0-X
A2	Split squat with dumbbells	12	3-0-X
A3	Step-up (with or without weight)	25	2-0-X
	REST 2 MINUTES. REPEAT 1 TO 5 MORE TIMES		
B1	Dumbbell dead lift	6	4-0-X
B2	Leg curl with stability ball	12	3-0-X
B3	Standing calf raise	25	2-0-X
	REST 2 MINUTES. REPEAT 1 TO 5 MORE TIMES		

Workout 4

	CHEST AND BACK	# REPS	TEMPO
A1	Flat bench dumbbell chest press	6	4-0-X
A2	Dumbbell pullover	12	3-0-X
A3	Incline dumbbell fly	25	2-0-X
	REST 2 MINUTES. REPEAT 1 TO 5 MORE TIMES		
B1	Pull-up	6	4-0-X
B2	Barbell reverse grip bent-over row	12	3-0-X
B3	Incline bench prone dumbbell row	25	2-0-X
	REST 2 MINUTES. REPEAT 1 TO 5 MORE TIMES		

Make sure to incorporate four workouts and three rest days in a seven-day period and then repeat the training cycle, starting with Workout 1.

BECOME A BODY SCULPTOR: HOW TO COAX STUBBORN BODY PARTS TO GROW

I can recall seeing a hilarious commercial on television advertising the merits of training at a particular gym. In the commercial, a huge and very defined bodybuilder responds to every question the gym owner asks, and then some, by saying, "I pick things up and put them down."

If only things were that simple.

Most trainees make the mistake of thinking all that is required to stimulate muscle growth is moving a weight from point A to point B. Granted, this is what power lifters do, but this is not the way of the body sculptor. To be a true body sculptor, you must focus on creating maximal amounts of *tension* in the muscle.

Tension is how hard a muscle is being targeted during an exercise. An increase in tension in a muscle amplifies the amount of damage imposed, leading to a greater degree of protein degradation and, ultimately, muscle growth. Heavy-weight training in the 1 to 3 rep range provides the greatest amount of tension. But there is a problem with this scenario: the time a muscle is under tension is insufficient to produce maximal muscle growth. This is the main reason lifting heavy for low reps is best for people looking to increase strength without increasing muscle size.

However, when coaxing a stubborn body part to grow, you will need to focus on increasing the amount of *time* the targeted muscle is under tension. By increasing "time under tension," or TUT, you effectively create the ideal hormonal environment to bring about muscle growth.

There are many techniques you can use to increase TUT and bring up a stubborn body part, but perhaps the best is the highly effective method known as a "drop set." With this technique, you perform a set of any exercise to failure or just short of failure, then drop some weight and continue for more repetitions with the reduced load. Drop sets are great for increasing muscle size and are generally not used for any other purpose.

How to Do a Drop Set

Drop sets, also known as "running the rack," are excellent for targeting virtually any stubborn body part and can be performed using most types of fitness equipment. Let's use dumbbells as an example. Simply start by choosing an exercise for the body part you want to target and select your starting weight. Perform 6 to 8 reps with this weight and then grab the next lower dumbbell weight and perform another 6 to 8 reps of the same exercise. This can be repeated for up to four "drops" in weight. For example, if you start doing squats with two 30-pound dumbbells, you will drop to 25, 20 and 15 for a complete set.

You can incorporate this technique into the 6-12-25 Protocol by picking an isolation exercise that targets your stubborn body part and performing 2 to 3 drop sets for it. You can do this at the beginning or end of your workout—it is up to you. Flex as hard as possible during every portion of the lift, and never allow the tension to diminish for the duration of each set. I recommend picking one or two body parts per workout, and applying this technique to that body part no more often than two to three times per week. For example, if you want to improve your biceps, incorporate 1 or 2 drop sets of bicep curls after Workout 3, the lower-body workout.

Smile . . . and enjoy the pain. It will be worth it in the end.

11

Sexy on Demand

How to Peak for a Special Event

I often receive requests to outline a game plan for people who are in great shape but want to take it to the next level and get in what I call "special-event shape." This program isn't aimed at people with a lot of fat to lose; rather, it is the perfect program for a person who is in excellent shape and wants to take it a step up to their most ideal body shape.

For example, I judge my condition by how visible my abdominal muscles are, and most of the year I stay in quite good shape, with some visible abdominal definition. In terms of percent body fat, my typical measurement is between 9% and 10%. Occasionally, there are times when this "good" isn't good enough for me and I want to take my condition up a notch and drop my body fat down to 6% or 7%. (I usually do this about once per year, and that's as often as I would recommend anyone else do it as well.) Women, however, should not take their body fat so low and would therefore use the program to reduce their body fat percentage to the 12% to 15% range.

The methods you are about to learn might be considered rather extreme, but remember, they are not meant to be followed year-round. In fact, I have designed this program to be used for a four-week period maximum. It's strictly for those instances when you absolutely, positively need to look your best for a special event. A healthy person can be pushed hard for a short period, and that's what this program is designed to do. One disclaimer: *do not* implement the following techniques if you have more than 5 to 10 pounds (max) to lose *or* if you have any health problems. Do this program only if you are in very good shape already and have a solid foundation of proper training, nutrition, and supplementation. I say this because I just know that some folks are going to buy this book and skip right to this chapter. If this is you, then stop, go back and read the book from the beginning, and implement those strategies first. *Doing otherwise will not produce the desired result.* So, if you are ready, let's get at it, shall we?

FOCUS ON WHAT MATTERS MOST

To get something you have never had, you are going to have to do something you have never done. The process of going from being in good shape to "Holy crap, you look *awesome!*" will require you working harder than you are accustomed to. I am about to take you out of your comfort zone and over to a place you are not going to love. Remember, this is only temporary and not intended to be followed for the long term. During this phase, you'll focus on one thing and one thing only: getting your body looking ultra-sexy in the shortest time possible. The first and most important part of this process is your diet. The goal of this program is to temporarily throw your body into a severe calorie deficit while simultaneously exercising to pre-serve lean muscle mass.

To calculate how many calories you will be eating daily for the next four weeks, use this formula:

Your body weight in pounds × 8 kcal = number of calories per day

For example, let's say you are a woman who weighs 140 pounds. Your daily calorie allotment would be 1120: 140 × 8 = 1120. The chart below illustrates a few calculations, allowing for a 10% variable plus or minus.

Special-Event Fat-Loss Calorie Guide

BODY WEIGHT	DAILY CALORIE INTAKE (−/+ 10% RANGE)
100 lb	800 kcal (720–880 kcal)
150 lb	1200 kcal (1080–1320 kcal)
200 lb	1600 kcal (1440–1760 kcal)
250 lb	2000 kcal (1800–2200 kcal)
300 lb	2400 kcal (2160–2640 kcal)

Yes, this is low, but remember, this is temporary. You will continue this cycle for up to four weeks (after which you will have reached your goal and should switch over to the program outlined in chapter 10).

During this program, I recommend that you follow a meal plan. Here is how to break things down.

MACRONUTRIENTS: PROTEINS, CARBOHYDRATES, AND FATS

Protein

Protein will be relatively high and will make up approximately 40% of your total daily calories. Protein is critical during a low-calorie diet in order to keep the feeling of hunger under control and to preserve lean muscle mass. Protein is also "thermic," costing your body energy in its digestion. During this phase, focus on consuming whole foods in addition to some supplements. Please don't live off protein shakes—whole-food protein sources will provide more bang for your buck in terms of nutrients and satiety. It's okay to use protein shakes during this program (and you will see them included below), but I don't want you to subsist on them.

Carbohydrates

Carbohydrates are going to be cut big time. For the duration of this program, your carbs should be no higher than 20% of total calories *max*. In addition, *all* carbs must come from vegetable sources, with the emphasis being on those with the greatest nutrient density, such as kale, broccoli, spinach, green beans, asparagus, zucchini, and peppers. I also like to include some fermented foods—don't shy away from things like sauerkraut. Try to buy organic vegetables whenever possible and make sure to wash them thoroughly before eating.

Fats

Fats will make up the balance of your calories and should come in at about 40% of total calories. Try to minimize your intake of omega-6 oils (such as canola) and focus on consuming omega-3, -7, and -9 from a variety of sources, including fish, flaxseed, olives, macadamias, coconuts, krill, and avocados.

WHEN TO EAT

I discussed meal frequency in chapter 5. As mentioned there, what matters most is total calories consumed for the day, *not* how those calories are dispersed. When calories are quite low (as they are with this program), frequent feeding becomes problematic because of how small the meals have to be. The strategy of five or six small meals per day seems to work best for larger, more active individuals whose daily calorie requirements can allow for eating small meals that still have some substance to them. For women who need to follow a 1200-calorie diet, eating six 200-calorie "meals" just seems ludicrous. For that reason I want you to eat in the way that works best for you. If you prefer to eat three meals per day, go for it. Want to stretch those calories out to five meals per day? No problem. Just remember that you must adhere to your daily calorie limits in order for this program to work.

SUPPLEMENTS

Because of the aggressive calorie cutting involved in this program, you run the risk of nutrient deficiencies and muscle loss. And when you combine a low-calorie diet with lots of exercise, it's pretty well guaranteed that some nutrient gaps will need to be filled. At this time, supplementation increases in importance and will go a long way to keeping you performing well and feeling as "normal" as can be expected. For this reason, it is imperative that you incorporate the Tier 1 and Tier 2 supplements discussed in chapter 9, as well as the fat-burning supplements abs+, which contains EGCG and CLA, and lean+, which contains Coleus forskohlii, HCA, and ALA (see chapter 9 for more on these ingredients). If you do not have access to these supplements, be sure to choose a fat burner that contains Coleus forskohlii. If cost is an issue, think of it this way: with this diet, you will be purchasing fewer groceries and avoiding restaurants, and this should more than make up for the costs incurred by buying additional supplements. Yes, you could do the program without them, but I promise that you will feel and perform a lot better if you simply bite the bullet and use them as outlined below.

WHEN TO BEGIN

The goal with this 4-week program is to have you looking your very best on a particular day. This could be your wedding, a beach vacation, high school reunion, or any event where you want to show off how great you look. Again, this is not intended as a long-term fat-loss program. Instead, it's a way to trick your body into ridding itself of subcutaneous water weight and fat in order to produce that nice dry look you see on swimsuit models and fitness competitors. For this to work, you will need to pick a target date for looking your best. From this date simply subtract four weeks and make that date your start date to begin the process.

WEEKS 1 TO 3

Nutrition

For this program to work, you will need to manipulate your sodium and water intake, so for the next three weeks you will be increasing both. Don't worry about an increase in sodium and any potential effect this may have on blood pressure. If you are at the recommended percent body fat when starting this program, blood pressure should not be an issue. Follow these nutrition guidelines for the next three weeks:

1. **Increase sodium intake.** Begin lightly salting your meals. Any type of salt will work, so don't worry if you don't have sea salt. Your goal is to consume approximately 20 milligrams of sodium for each pound of body weight (per day, not per meal).

2. **Increase water intake.** Start drinking a minimum of half your body weight in ounces of water each day.

3. **Consume only whole foods for your main meals.** No meal-replacement shakes are permitted.

4. **Keep protein intake high.** Women should consume 1 gram of protein per pound of body weight daily; men should consume 1.5 grams per pound of body weight daily.

5. **Consume 2 tablespoons (if female) or 3 tablespoons (if male) of healthy fats each day (not including the fish oil).** These fats can be coconut oil, extra-virgin olive oil, or butter from grass-fed cows, for instance. They can be used when cooking your meals or added after cooking.

6. **Consume a post-workout protein shake.** This should consist of 0.25 grams of protein per pound of body weight, 1 to 2 ounces of fruit juice of your choice, and 5 grams of creatine supplement (see shake recipe on page 185).

7. **Increase intake of fibrous carbohydrates.** The only carbs you are allowed to consume are green vegetables—none other.

Exercise

To hit your peak on a particular day, you are going to temporarily increase your training frequency. The goal is to deplete muscle glycogen and burn fat while still retaining as much lean muscle mass as possible. To do this you will need to do the following:

1. **Perform low-intensity cardio 6 days per week.** The benefits of low-intensity, long-duration cardio are amplified during a low-calorie phase. The cardio is to be performed first thing in the morning on an empty

stomach (my preference for you) *or* immediately post–weight-training workout. Progress your low-intensity cardio sessions as follows:

LOW-INTENSITY CARDIO PROGRESSION	
Week 1	30 minutes/6 days per week
Week 2	40 minutes/6 days per week
Week 3	50 minutes/6 days per week

2. **Exercise with resistance 4 days per week.** Weight training during this phase is for two purposes: muscle preservation and glycogen depletion. This is not a time that you will be building muscle mass or setting a new personal best. Here is the structure of your exercise program:

WEEKS 1 TO 3 EXERCISE STRUCTURE

Monday: Upper body
Perform Workout 4 from the 6-12-25 Protocol (page 202).

Tuesday: Lower body
Perform Workout 3 from the 6-12-25 Protocol (page 201).

Wednesday: Upper body
Perform Workout 2 from the 6-12-25 Protocol (page 201).

Thursday: Cardio only

Friday: Total body
Perform Protocol 3 (Friday workout) from page 149, and include the additional evening sprint workout.

Saturday: Cardio only

Sunday: Off

Diet

By now you are probably wondering what the diet will look like. Here's an example:

Upon Wake-Up

12 ounces water

One serving greens+ or other greens supplement

Multivitamin/multimineral

2 capsules fish oil

3 capsules abs+

2 capsules lean+

5 grams creatine

5 grams BCAAs

1 cup green tea

During Your Resistance-Training Workout

Sip 5 grams of BCAAs mixed in 4 cups of water. After your workout, drink your post-workout shake.

Breakfast

Omelet made with 3 organic whole eggs

1 cup chopped spinach

1 tablespoon salsa

½ cup sliced mushrooms

1 cup water

Lunch

1 medium serving homemade turkey chili (with celery, mushrooms, tomatoes, peppers, and zucchini)

1 cup water

3 capsules abs+

2 capsules lean+

2 capsules fish oil

Midday Snack (Optional)
> 5 grams BCAAs

The BCAAs are optional, but I find they work very well to calm any hunger pangs. You could also use 1 scoop of whey or vegetarian protein powder mixed in water; I recommend alternating between the two.

Dinner
> 1 medium serving protein source, such as beef, fish, or vegetable
> 1 cup water
> 3 capsules abs+
> 2 capsules lean+
> 2 capsules fish oil

You'll notice that dinner is similar to lunch—I like to keep things simple when cutting calories. It's best to use a different protein source, though.

Pre-Bed Snack (Optional)
> 5 grams BCAAs or 1 serving whey protein with a dash of cinnamon
> 2 capsules fish oil
> 1 serving magnesium (200 to 400 milligrams)

The pre-bed snack too is optional. I can't fall asleep when my stomach's grumbling, so I tend to have this.

The Finer Points of Weeks 1 to 3
The finer points of the first three weeks of this program can be summarized as follows:

1. **Go into every workout in a carbohydrate-fasted state.** Don't eat any fats or carbohydrates for at least three hours prior to exercise. The only food energy during this period should come from 5 to 10 grams of BCAAs. This is to ensure that your insulin levels are kept low and will allow for maximum release of growth hormone (great for fat burning).

2. **Know your calorie limit and stay within it.** During this period, it is absolutely essential to consume only foods that have a high nutrient density. You must follow a meal plan so that you know how many calories you are taking in. Foods like chicken breasts and vegetables will be the foundation of your nutrition plan. Alcohol is out for now (it offers no nutrient benefits). Resolve yourself to the notion that this is about getting your body to strip fat as fast as possible while retaining muscle mass. This means that your diet will need to be quite boring. Once you reach your goal, you will be able to loosen the reins and look hot eating and drinking the foods you love.

3. **Use supplements to fill nutrient gaps.** Supplements become more important as calories decrease and activity increases. This is the time when you will notice a significant difference in how you feel, perform, and look depending on the supplements you use. Protein supplementation in the form of BCAAs and whey and/ or vegetarian protein powders will help you feel fuller longer (and a whole lot less irritable during this time). Multivitamins, minerals, green drinks, and fish oils will fill nutrient gaps. Fat burners such as lean+ and abs+ will give your body a slight fat-burning boost.

4. **Increase sodium intake.** I know this point will be met with some resistance from the medical community and nutrition zealots, but keep in mind this program's

approach. We are trying to manipulate subcutaneous water retention, and to do so you will have to temporarily increase your sodium intake.

5. **Increase water consumption.** It seems counterintuitive, but drinking more water will help you eliminate more of the subcutaneous water retention that can make you appear fat and bloated. Consume half your body weight in ounces of water each day, and more on days you sweat a lot. I like to flavor my water with fresh lemon or lime juice, and this also helps improve the body's ability to consume such high amounts. It will be an inconvenience for a while (plan your bathroom breaks) but definitely worth it in the end.

6. **Exercise six days per week.** Your body can take the increase in exercise frequency for a short period. My preference is to perform four resistance-training sessions per week as outlined, *plus* daily low-intensity cardio sessions. Even walking is helpful during this period. This can be sustained for up to four weeks *max*, then take a week off completely from all diet and exercise routines.

7. **Consume protein around each workout.** Muscle catabolism is most likely to occur during periods of low-calorie and low-carbohydrate intake and increased exercise volume. You can minimize the chances of this by keeping protein intake high. The two critical periods are pre- and post-workout. Just be sure to not go crazy with the carbs.

8. **Restrict carbs.** I am far from being carb-phobic, but after testing it on numerous occasions, I can tell you that this plan works best when carbs are strictly controlled. Just to be clear, when I say "carbs," I am talking about foods such as potatoes, rice, breads,

oatmeal, pasta, quinoa, and grains. Fruit should also be kept to a bare minimum. You can eat all the cruciferous vegetable carbs your hungry heart desires.

WEEK 4: COUNTDOWN TO THE BIG DAY!

In this final week, you will be making some small but critical changes to both your diet and training program.

Nutrition

Monday, Tuesday, and Wednesday: Continue to eat as described in the Diet section for weeks 1 to 3 (pages 213–14) except remove all carbohydrates from your protein shakes and meals. Green veggies, protein, and fat *only*. No exceptions. Continue to keep fluid intake high, and lightly salt your meals.

Thursday: After your workout, begin carbohydrate loading. Your post-workout protein shake should contain between 75 and 100 grams of fast-digesting carbs such as maple syrup or malto-dextrin. Continue to eat lots of carbohydrates throughout the day—I recommend eating a carb-rich meal every two to three waking hours. Your goal is to consume approximately 3 grams of carbs per pound of body weight (if male) or 1.5 grams per pound (if female). Choose good-quality, clean carbs such as white rice, white or sweet potatoes, or gluten-free oats. Continue keeping fluid intake high and lightly salting your meals.

Friday: No workout today, and the carbohydrate party is over. Today you will remove the carbs, cease salting your foods, and eat protein and fats only. You must also start drinking lots of water early in the morning, with the goal of consuming 2 ounces per pound of body weight before 6 p.m., after which you will stop all eating and drinking.

Saturday: The *big* day. Today is your target date for looking your best, and if you have followed my advice, you will be looking damn good indeed! No training today, but you must eat a protein- and carbohydrate-rich breakfast. Some fat is fine too, but keep your water intake to a minimum. You can sip small amounts with your meals, but nothing more. Some people benefit in terms of muscles appearing fuller than they otherwise would from having some high-calorie foods such as pizza on this day, so don't be afraid to experiment with what works best for you. Be sure to take some pics of your awesome self, because you have earned it!

Exercise

To keep things simple, your training program in week 4 will remain the same as in weeks 1 to 3 except for these key points:

- Eliminate all cardio.
- Increase repetitions and decrease weight. Your goal is to perform between 40 and 50 reps per set.
- Substitute machines for free weights. This is an occasion when using machines may be the best choice as they require less balance and concentration. Performing high-rep workouts in a carb-depleted state using free weights can be very difficult. If you prefer, substitute squats for the leg press or leg extension, for example.

Structure your workouts in the final week as follows:

WEEK 4 EXERCISE STRUCTURE

Monday: Upper body
Perform Workout 4 from the 6-12-25 Protocol (page 202).

Tuesday: Lower body
Perform Workout 3 from the 6-12-25 Protocol (page 201).

Wednesday: Upper body
Perform Workout 2 from the 6-12-25 Protocol (page 201).

Thursday: Total body
Perform Protocol 3 (Friday workout) from page 149 and include the additional evening sprint workout.

Friday: Off

Saturday: Off

If you make it through this, you are a true champion! Be sure to send me the pics!

12

The Trouble Spot Maintenance Plan

These days, we are all busy with our jobs, families, and friends, and finding the time to take care of ourselves often takes a back seat to other priorities. With this in mind, the *Trouble Spot Fat Loss* nutrition and training protocols are not meant to be followed forever. They are meant as go-to strategies for losing those last pounds and inches that you cannot lose no matter what you try.

I know that following the program wasn't easy, and I know that you made some sacrifices along the way. But I have good news for you. You now know more about how to transform your body than does 99% of the world's population. Congratulations—you are officially an "expert"! But before you go getting a swelled head, I want to tell you something a very successful client once told me: it is one thing to achieve a certain level of success; it's another thing to hold on to it. Fortunately, when it comes to trouble spot fat, once you have lost it, keeping it off is actually quite simple. The Trouble Spot Maintenance Plan consists of a simple daily to-do list for maintaining those awesome results (while having a life). Implement the plan and keep that trouble spot fat off for the long term.

The Trouble Spot Fat Loss program introduced you to a number of new behaviors in terms of how you spend your time, and these will have created a result. Going forward, focus on forming a few habits for your mind, body, and diet. Repeat them each day and soon they will become the daily routines that will successfully keep you lean, muscular, strong, and fit for the rest of your life.

MIND

Adopting the right mind-set is essential to achieving success and avoiding regression.

Do Something Each Day That Supports Your Goals

Mark Twain once said, "Twenty years from now, you will be more disappointed by the things you didn't do than by the ones you did. So throw off the bowlines. Sail away from the safe harbor. Catch the trade winds in your sails. Explore. Dream. Discover." Do not be the person who wishes for things to happen to them. Be the person who makes things happen for themselves. Take action each day by implementing at least one thing that supports your goal of continued health and fitness.

Schedule Your Success

Take 15 minutes each evening to outline your perfect day tomorrow. Plan when you are going to wake up, what you are going to eat, and when you are going to train. Try to include a combination of work, fun, family, and exercise. Focus on quality of time spent and not just quantity. Success is something we must plan for.

Always Keep the Goal Top of Mind

It is very easy to get discouraged and fall off the track of eating well and training consistently. It happens at each New Year. Hordes of people start exercising and eating healthy, only to eventually return to their old ways. It is almost as if they forgot why they started exercising and eating healthy in the first place. I remind myself *daily* about the person I want to be. Put up pictures, notes, and other reminders in places where you have to look at them. I have used this technique for two decades and it helps keep me focused on what I truly desire.

Accept That You Are on Your Own

Nobody else can do this for you. There is no easy way out. You simply have to dig in your heels and accept the fact that your body and how it looks and performs is up to you. Drop the excuses and just do it already.

Surround Yourself with Like-Minded, Success-Oriented People

Whenever I am around someone who has accomplished extraordinary things, I cannot help but be inspired to achieve more. If you're hanging out with people who are doing what you want to do, you'll start to adopt their habits. If your friends are keeping you up late drinking and eating crap, then it may be time for some new ones. The right social circle can provide you with support, encouragement, and mentorship. You will end up accomplishing your goals quicker because you'll be in an environment that supports it.

Stop Wasting Time

Each one of us has been assigned a finite and unknown amount of time on this planet, and each day millions of us piss away valuable minutes and hours doing meaningless, stupid, and often self-destructive stuff. News flash: you are going to die, and the clock is ticking. Legendary marketer Dan Kennedy has a clock in his home that is counting down to his estimated expiration date. Talk about a daily reminder of how valuable your time really is. Whatever it is that you want to accomplish, do it now.

BODY

Your body was made to move, and training, sweating, and exercising your body on a consistent basis just plain makes sense (and feels good). It releases endorphins and strengthens bones, while building and maintaining muscle mass. You don't have to live in a gym in order to look great the whole year round. You will be surprised (and happy) to discover how little exercise is necessary to maintain results.

Exercise a Minimum of Three Times per Week

Once you have achieved your fat-loss or muscle-building goal, maintenance can be achieved simply by subjecting your major muscle groups to some heavy resistance each week (to prevent atrophy). Light weights are not going to do the job. There is a saying in bodybuilding, "Whatever built the muscle will keep the muscle," and there is truth to it. You can do less volume of work, but you should still be working hard and lifting challenging loads. For many people, cardio can be reduced or even eliminated during a maintenance phase (as long as the diet is kept in check. If you have a carb orgy every day, you will pay for it).

Focus on Compound Movements

Compound movements like squats, dead lifts, and presses are better than isolation exercises like bicep curls and lateral raises, simply because they work more muscle and allow you to lift greater loads. Lifting heavy weights results in a more favorable hormonal response, and this in turn will help preserve your gains with fewer exercise sessions. Performing any workout that focuses just on the abs, say, will not have the same effect.

Always Warm Up

I have never sustained an injury during a workout for which I was properly warmed up. Always perform some mobility and flexibility movements to prepare your body for the work to come. Never jump directly into your heaviest set. Always perform a couple of low-rep, moderate-weight sets to prime your nervous system for the heavier work ahead.

Work Out Hard, Not Long

I estimate that less than 5% of the people at your local gym are actually training hard enough to accomplish their goals. Most people amble about with no defined plan and simply go through the motions. This never produces good results. Remember, gym time is work time. I think of it as going to war, and I want to win! Get focused and stop all the wandering to and from the water fountain and mindless chitchat. Effort equals reward, and nowhere else is this more evident than at the gym.

Perform Exercises You Hate

Most people repeat the same workout day in and day out and never do any of the exercises they hate. These exercises are inevitably the hardest and often include squats, unilateral movements, and hard-core intervals. These happen to be fantastic exercises for burning calories, building muscle, and maintaining a great body. Avoiding them will only leave you more susceptible to muscle imbalances, injury, and looking like a total wimp at the gym.

Always Try to Go One Better

Your body loves a challenge (even if you don't). If you fail to challenge your body, it will never change. Even in maintenance mode, it is still a good idea to try to "one up" yourself from time to time. This could be as simple as performing an extra repetition, sprinting an extra round, or adding 2 pounds to the bar. It will go a long way toward keeping the body you have worked so hard to obtain.

DIET

Diet will always be the single most significant (and difficult) barrier to long-term success. The secret is to keep things realistic and actionable. This can be accomplished by following these simple rules.

Focus on Nutrients Rather Than Calories

Calories matter, but once you move beyond a fat-burning or muscle-building phase, you can forget all about them and switch to focusing on nutrients instead. When you focus on consuming mostly nutrient-dense foods such as lean proteins, vegetables, and healthy fats, you will discover that maintaining your results is a breeze. All that you have to do is keep an eye on your current level of conditioning and not allow yourself to stray too far from it. If you do find yourself slipping, you can easily cut back a bit on your intake and pull yourself back from the edge.

Earn Your Carbs

This trick has had the single biggest impact on my ability to remain lean and muscular year-round. I simply do not eat any starchy carbs such as potatoes, rice, and bread unless I have exercised and earned the right to do so. On days that my activity level is low, I stick to eating proteins, veggies, and healthy fats. This works to keep both hunger and body fat under control.

Eat Real Food

There are hundreds of meal-replacement shakes and bars on the market, and the thrust of their marketing is that consuming them will provide some sort of metabolic benefit that surpasses eating the equivalent in whole food form. This is pure BS. I can recall a client telling me how the latest protein bar magically transforms any subsequent calories eaten into muscle rather than fat. And how a magical fairy dust you sprinkle on your food renders the calories eaten inert. All this is marketing-driven fantasy. Humans will always function best when given a diet consisting of real food, such as lean meat, vegetables, nuts, beans, and fruits—not food that comes packaged with a bar code.

Avoid Obesogens

All of the foods we consume are connected in one way or another to the soil. Synthetic fertilizers upset the soil's delicate balance, and this impacts the quality of food that is produced. Many of the chemicals used in food production are known to disrupt the human endocrine system and are classified as obesogens. These foreign chemical compounds are known to—

- Encourage the body to store fat and reprogram cells to become fat cells.
- Prompt the liver to become insulin resistant.
- Prevent leptin from being released from your fat cells to tell your body you are full.

Avoiding obesogens is possible and doesn't require you to turn your life upside down. Here's how to do it:

- Buy wild fish and grass-fed meat and dairy products that are hormone- and antibiotic-free.
- Install a granular-activated carbon filter on your faucet.
- Use stainless-steel, glass, or otherwise BPA-free water bottles.
- Avoid using food containers that contain BPA.
- Choose organic fruits and veggies whenever possible, and always wash thoroughly before consuming.
- Never microwave food in plastic.
- Eat fewer canned foods. Tuna can be found in pouches that do not contain harmful BPA.
- Get rid of your nonstick pans, if possible, as the coating contains toxics that can be released at high heat. Never used a scratched Teflon pan (use a wooden implement on it to avoid scratching).
- Buy meats straight from the butcher, and ask that it be wrapped in brown paper rather than plastic.
- Skip the air fresheners—open the windows, and try scenting the air with a vase of dried lavender instead.

Eat More Protein

If you've read this book through, the eat-more-protein rule will come as no surprise. I have found that the simple act of increasing protein consumption is often enough to bring about significant changes to body composition through a reduction in appetite and an increase in thermogenesis. To maintain your results, you don't have to obsess over the exact amount of protein to consume each day, just make sure that each time you eat, you include a good-quality protein from an animal or vegetable source.

Eat Fewer Processed Foods

This is a no-brainer. Processed carbohydrate foods like breads, cereals, pastas, rolls, crackers, cakes, candies, and fast foods are easily converted to sugar and extra body fat. Processed carbohydrates are the number one reason people are getting so fat these days. These foods are simply too calorie-dense and nutrient-sparse to be a part of your everyday lifestyle. Sure, it's okay to eat them on occasion, but always time their consumption to coincide with the post-exercise training period. In other words, you must earn the right to eat this crap.

Drink More Water and Tea

Your body is more than 80% water, so it makes good sense to keep well hydrated. Stay away from artificially sweetened water; instead, stick to drinking water with fresh-squeezed lemon or lime juice. Drink more on days you exercise or perspire heavily, and try not to drink excessive amounts with your meals as this can impede digestion. Teas are also great to have anytime, but try to keep coffee to the pre-workout period only.

Eat More Veggies

Veggies are often classified as "negative calorie" foods, as they can cost more energy to digest than they contain. Veggies are packed with nutrients and will help fill your plate (and stomach) without adding to your calorie load. Just keep them away from the deep fryer and season them using lemon juice and/or spices only, plus a little bit of sea salt, if you must.

Plan to Cheat

Life is not about deprivation, it's about earning your rewards. I always recommend scheduling diet breaks. Going too long without them can actually hinder your results. Plan when you are going to cheat, and enjoy every minute of the experience.

Recipes

ANYTIME MEALS

Anytime Meals are just that, meals that are great to eat at any time, whether you are in a fat-loss phase or not, pre-workout or post-workout. These meals are rich in the essential components of a fat-loss diet while being low in starch-based and refined carbohydrates. By reducing your intake of these carbohydrate foods, you are allowing for a natural inhibition of your body's alpha receptors and so improving the release and burning of fat from your stubborn fat cells. These meals will also improve satiety—a key factor for *sustainable* calorie reduction.

The Anytime Meals recipes contain each of the following three ingredients:

1. A protein selection
2. A fibrous vegetable selection
3. A fat selection

I have included calorie and nutrition information with each recipe, but, as you now know, calories should not be your primary focus. The important thing to keep in mind with both the Anytime and Post-Workout Meals is getting the right mix of macronutrients—proteins, fats, and carbs—for the fat-loss and muscle-building regimes. Keep your carbs low during a fat-loss phase, and when you are building muscle, make carbs a part of your post-workout diet.

To make preparation easy, the recipes with beans call for canned beans. Using dried beans and soaking is a better method for getting all the nutrients out of your food and avoiding potential BPA in cans. If you do used dried beans, use approximately half the specified amount in dried beans and reserve the cooking liquid when bean liquid is called for in the recipe (for example, with Black Bean Chili, page 238).

When preparing the meals, I also recommend that you—

- Favor coconut or avocado oils for cooking, they are less sensitive to heat than olive oil. But there are times when olive oil may be preferred, for example when medium or low heat is used for cooking, or when no heat is being used at all.
- Add spices according to your taste (all spices are okay to use).
- Try to stick with unrefined sea salt if using salt.

Most people plan their meals based on their food preferences. I often keep a simple salad dressing on hand to add extra flavor to an Anytime Meal. On the following page is a quick-and-easy recipe.

Everyday Vinaigrette

2 tablespoons red wine vinegar
   or apple cider vinegar

1 teaspoon Dijon mustard

½ cup extra-virgin olive oil

1 tablespoon flaxseed oil

Chopped fresh herbs of your
   choice (optional)

Place vinegar and mustard in a bowl and whisk to combine. Add olive oil and whisk until oil is well mixed or emulsified. Add flaxseed oil and fresh herbs, if using. Dressing will keep in the refrigerator, in a sealed container, for up to 3 days.

BREAKFAST

Fresh Herb Omelet

GLUTEN-FREE, SOY-FREE, DAIRY-FREE, VEGETARIAN

Serves 4

Per serving: 190 calories, 8 g fat, 3 g carbohydrate, 1 g fiber, 15 g protein

3 tablespoons avocado oil,
   divided

1 large red or white onion,
   chopped

1 bunch Swiss chard or spinach,
   leaves only, chopped

Sea salt and freshly ground black
   pepper

1 garlic clove

6 to 8 eggs

2 tablespoons chopped fresh
   parsley

2 tablespoons chopped fresh basil

2 teaspoons chopped fresh thyme

In a large frying pan, heat 2 tablespoons oil over medium-high heat. Add onion, reduce heat to low, and cook for 15 minutes, until soft. Add Swiss chard and cook, stirring occasionally, until all the moisture has evaporated and chard is tender, about 15 minutes. Transfer mixture to a large bowl. Season with sea salt and pepper.

Meanwhile, lightly beat eggs in a large bowl. Crush garlic and add a few pinches of sea salt (or finely chop them together), then stir into eggs, along with herbs. Add chard mixture to egg mixture, stirring to combine.

Heat the remaining 1 tablespoon oil in the frying pan over medium-high heat, then add egg mixture. Give it a stir, keeping heat at medium-high for about 1 minute before reducing to low. Cook until egg mixture is set but still a little moist on top, 10 to 15 minutes.

Berry Yogurt

GLUTEN-FREE, SOY-FREE, VEGETARIAN

Serves 1

Per serving: 150 calories, 7 g fat, 6 g carbohydrate, 1 g fiber, 15 g protein

⅓ cup blueberries   ¾ cup plain Greek yogurt

Mix blueberries into yogurt and enjoy.

Seedy Cereal

GLUTEN-FREE, SOY-FREE, DAIRY-FREE, VEGAN

Serves 1

Per serving: 160 calories, 10 g fat, 15 g carbohydrate, 9 g fiber, 20 g protein

½ cup unsweetened hemp or coconut milk

1 ½ scoops vanilla protein powder (vegan or whey)

12 blueberries

6 raspberries

3 strawberries, sliced

1 tablespoon chia seeds

1 tablespoon organic hulled hemp seeds

½ tablespoon organic buckwheat

In a shaker cup, shake together hemp milk and protein powder to combine.

Place berries in a bowl. Pour shake over berries and sprinkle chia and hemp seeds, along with buckwheat, over top. Let stand for 5 minutes to allow seeds to expand. Serve and enjoy.

LUNCH

Turkey Lettuce Wraps

GLUTEN-FREE, DAIRY-FREE

Serves 4

Per serving: 300 calories, 18 g fat, 7 g carbohydrate, 3 g fiber, 32 g protein

1 tablespoon coconut oil

1 large onion, chopped

1¼ pounds lean ground turkey

½ cup peanut sauce

1 tablespoon hoisin sauce

1 tablespoon gluten-free soy sauce + extra for dipping

1 cucumber, peeled and chopped

⅓ cup chopped fresh mint + ⅓ cup small fresh mint sprigs

Sea salt and freshly ground black pepper

12 large butter lettuce leaves

In a large frying pan, heat coconut oil over medium-high heat. Add onion and sauté for 3 minutes or until beginning to brown. Add turkey and sauté for 7 minutes or until brown and cooked through. Add peanut sauce, hoisin sauce, and soy sauce. Stir in cucumber and chopped mint. Season with sea salt and pepper. Transfer turkey mixture to a medium bowl.

Arrange mint sprigs and lettuce leaves on a platter. To make wraps, spoon some turkey mixture onto a lettuce leaf, add a few mint sprigs, then fold in one side of lettuce over filling and roll up. Serve soy sauce alongside wraps for dipping.

TIP: For this, and other like low-carb meals, lettuce works as an excellent substitute for tortillas or rice wraps.

Ginger Shrimp Stir-Fry

GLUTEN-FREE, SOY-FREE, DAIRY-FREE

Serves 4

Per serving: 275 calories, 9 g fat, 16 g carbohydrate, 5 g fiber, 28 g protein

1 pound uncooked large shrimp, peeled and deveined

2 tablespoons coconut oil, divided

2 large garlic cloves, minced, divided

3 teaspoons peeled and minced fresh ginger, divided

½ teaspoon sea salt

¼ teaspoon dried crushed red pepper

1 pound sugar snap peas, strings removed

1 zucchini, thinly sliced

½ cup diced red bell pepper

3 green onions, thinly sliced

Sea salt and freshly ground black pepper

2 teaspoons black or white sesame seeds (optional)

In a medium bowl, mix shrimp, 1 tablespoon oil, half of the garlic, 1½ teaspoons ginger, sea salt, and crushed red pepper.

Heat a large frying pan over high heat. Sauté shrimp mixture until shrimp are cooked through, about 2 minutes. Transfer to the bowl. Add the remaining 1 tablespoon oil to the frying pan, then add snap peas, zucchini, bell pepper, green onions, the remaining 1½ teaspoons ginger, and the remaining garlic. Stir-fry for 3 minutes or until vegetables are crisp-tender.

Return shrimp mixture to the frying pan and stir-fry for 1 minute. Season with sea salt and pepper, sprinkle with sesame seeds, if using, and serve.

Spiced Steak Salad

GLUTEN-FREE, SOY-FREE, DAIRY-FREE

Serves 4

Per serving: 275 calories, 20 g fat, 12 g carbohydrate, 4 g fiber, 15 g protein

SPICE RUB

½ tablespoon paprika

2 teaspoons ground black pepper

1½ teaspoons sea salt

1 teaspoon garlic powder

1 teaspoon cayenne pepper

½ teaspoon dried oregano

½ teaspoon dried thyme

DRESSING

¼ cup extra-virgin olive oil

2½ tablespoons balsamic vinegar

1 tablespoon chopped fresh basil

1 teaspoon Dijon mustard

Sea salt and freshly ground black pepper

SALAD

6 cups organic mixed baby greens

½ red bell pepper, thinly sliced

½ cup thinly sliced onion

2 6-ounce beef tenderloin steaks, each about ½ inch thick

3 tablespoons coconut butter, melted

1 tomato, quartered

Mix all spice rub ingredients together in a small bowl.

For the dressing, whisk together olive oil, balsamic vinegar, basil, and mustard in a small bowl. Season with sea salt and pepper.

For the salad, toss together greens, bell pepper, and onion in a large bowl. Add dressing to taste and toss. Divide salad between 4 plates.

Spread spice rub on a plate. Coat both sides of steaks with coconut butter, then press both sides into rub. Heat a large frying pan over high heat. Add steaks and cook for 2 minutes per side for medium-rare, or until cooked through (your preference). Transfer to a cutting board and let stand for 2 minutes. Thinly slice steaks crosswise. Arrange slices atop plated salad. Garnish with tomato.

DINNER

Roasted Salmon and Green Beans

GLUTEN-FREE, SOY-FREE, DAIRY-FREE

Serves 4

Per serving: 292 calories, 19 g fat, 5 g carbohydrate, 2 g fiber, 25 g protein

SALMON

1 teaspoon paprika

1 teaspoon garlic powder

1 teaspoon sea salt

½ teaspoon ground black pepper

Zest and juice of 1 lemon

1 tablespoon avocado oil

1 wild salmon fillet (about 2½ pounds)

GREEN BEANS

1 pound green beans, trimmed

3 garlic cloves, minced

1 tablespoon avocado oil

1 teaspoon sea salt

¼ cup chopped almonds

Preheat the oven to 400°F. Line a baking pan with foil.

In a small bowl, mix together paprika, garlic powder, sea salt, pepper, and lemon zest. Add avocado oil and mix well. Set salmon on the prepared pan. Gently rub the seasoning mixture over top of salmon. Set aside.

In a medium bowl, toss green beans with garlic, avocado oil, and sea salt. Arrange beans around salmon. Roast for 25 minutes or until fish flakes easily when tested with a fork. Sprinkle beans with almonds, drizzle lemon juice over salmon, and serve.

Black Bean Chili

GLUTEN-FREE, SOY-FREE, DAIRY-FREE, VEGAN

Serves 8

Per serving: 240 calories, 5 g fat, 25 g carbohydrate, 6 g fiber, 10 g protein

¼ cup coconut oil

2 cups chopped onion

1²/₃ cups coarsely chopped red bell pepper

6 garlic cloves, chopped

2 tablespoons chili powder

2 teaspoons dried oregano

1 ½ teaspoons ground cumin

½ teaspoon cayenne pepper

½ teaspoon turmeric

1 16-ounce can tomato sauce

3 15-ounce cans black beans, drained and rinsed, ½ cup liquid reserved

Sea salt and freshly ground black pepper

Chopped fresh cilantro

Chopped green onions

Heat oil in a large pot over medium-high heat. Add onion, bell pepper, and garlic. Sauté until onion softens, about 10 minutes. Add chili powder, oregano, cumin, cayenne, and turmeric, and cook, stirring, for 2 minutes. Stir in tomato sauce, beans, and reserved bean liquid. Bring chili to a boil, stirring occasionally. Reduce heat to medium-low and simmer, stirring occasionally, until flavors blend and mixture thickens. Season with sea salt and pepper.

Serve chili in individual bowls, topped with cilantro and green onions.

Zucchini Noodles with Meatballs

GLUTEN-FREE, SOY-FREE, DAIRY-FREE

Serves 3

Per serving: 325 calories, 15 g fat, 15 g carbohydrate, 7 g fiber, 25 g protein

MEATBALLS

2 garlic cloves, roughly chopped

1 small onion, roughly chopped

1/2 cup packed arugula or spinach leaves

1/3 cup fresh parsley, roughly chopped

8 fresh sage leaves

8 large fresh basil leaves

4 sprigs fresh thyme, leaves only

1 large sprig fresh rosemary, leaves only

1 teaspoon sea salt

1/2 teaspoon ground black pepper

1 pound ground turkey

2 cups sugar-free marinara sauce

1/4 cup water

ZUCCHINI NOODLES

1 tablespoon extra-virgin olive oil

1/4 cup diced red onion

3 garlic cloves, minced

3 zucchini, cut into long julienne strips

Sea salt and freshly ground black pepper

For the meatballs, place garlic, onion, arugula, herbs, sea salt, and pepper in a food processor and process until finely chopped. Using your hands or a fork, thoroughly combine mixture with turkey in a mixing bowl. Roll into 12 balls, each approximately the size of a golf ball.

Preheat the oven to 375°F. Place meatballs directly on a rimmed baking sheet. Bake for 20 minutes.

For the zucchini noodles, heat a large frying pan over medium heat. Add oil, onion, and garlic and cook for 1 to 2 minutes. Increase heat to medium-high and add zucchini. Season with sea salt and pepper, and cook, stirring, for 2 to 2½ minutes, until vegetables are warmed through yet still firm.

Before serving, mix marinara sauce with water in a medium saucepan. Add meatballs and stir gently to coat with sauce. Cover and simmer over low heat for 5 minutes.

Divide noodles between 3 bowls and top each with 4 meatballs and sauce.

SNACKS

Protein Nut Bars

GLUTEN-FREE, SOY-FREE, DAIRY-FREE, VEGETARIAN

Serves 6

Per serving: 379 calories, 20 g fat, 10 g carbohydrate, 4 g fiber, 30 g protein

1 cup almond flour

⅓ cup coconut flour

¼ cup walnut pieces

2 omega-3 eggs

2 egg whites, beaten

6 scoops vanilla protein powder (vegan or whey)

¼ teaspoon sea salt

Stevia, to taste

Coconut or olive oil

Preheat the oven to 350°F.

Mix all ingredients together in a large bowl, stirring to combine. Spread dough in a large baking dish coated with oil and bake for 15 minutes. Remove from oven and allow to cool before cutting slab into individual bars. Store in fridge in an airtight container.

Chocolate Protein Pudding

GLUTEN-FREE, SOY-FREE, VEGETARIAN

Serves 1

Per serving: 360 calories, 16 g fat, 14 g carbohydrate, 5 g fiber, 40 g protein

½ cup low-fat cottage cheese (preferably organic)

2 tablespoons flax meal

1 tablespoon almond or peanut butter

1 scoop chocolate whey protein powder

Stevia, to taste (optional)

Mix together all ingredients in a bowl, or process in a blender for a smooth and creamy texture.

Almond Butter Bars

GLUTEN-FREE, SOY-FREE, DAIRY-FREE, VEGAN

Serves 4

Per serving: 280 calories, 15 g fat, 10 g carbohydrate, 6 g fiber, 30 g protein

4 scoops chocolate protein powder (vegan or whey)

⅔ cup flax meal or ground chia seeds

4 tablespoons chunky almond butter

¼ cup filtered water

Stevia, to taste

Mix together all ingredients in a large bowl. Add more water if mixture is too dry. Shape mixture into separate bars. Chill and store bars in the fridge or freezer using an airtight container.

POST-WORKOUT MEALS

Post-Workout Meals differ from Anytime Meals in that they contain higher amounts of starch-based carbohydrates. These carbs help replenish muscle glycogen lost through exercise, boost leptin levels, and spike insulin, an important anabolic, or tissue-building, hormone.

These meals are best consumed after your resistance-training workout, during a muscle-building phase. Alternatively, they may be consumed on "cheat" days (see chapter 4) during a fat-loss phase.

Post-Workout Meal recipes consist of three main types of ingredients:

1. A protein selection
2. A vegetable selection
3. A starchy-carbohydrate selection

Your Post-Workout Meal may be eaten at any time of day. Just try to consume this meal *after* completing your muscle-building workout.

BREAKFAST

Blueberry Protein Pancakes

GLUTEN-FREE, SOY-FREE, DAIRY-FREE, VEGETARIAN

Serves 2 (makes 4 large pancakes)
Per serving (*without topping*): 240 calories, 5 g fat, 20 g carbohydrate, 5 g fiber, 30 g protein

½ small ripe banana

2 egg whites

2 teaspoons cinnamon

1 scoop protein powder (vegan or whey non-flavoured or vanilla)

¼ cup blueberries

½ cup unsweetened almond milk

In a bowl, mash banana into a paste. Stir in egg whites, sprinkle in cinnamon, add protein powder and blueberries, and then pour in almond milk. Stir together.

Ladle one-quarter of the batter onto a preheated greased griddle or into a frying pan set over medium heat and cook until the pancake bottom is golden and air bubbles form on the top, about 2½ minutes. Flip and cook on the other side, about another 2½ minutes. Transfer to a 250°F oven to keep warm while you cook the remaining 3 pancakes.

Serve topped with maple syrup and extra blueberries.

244 • BRUCE KRAHN

High-Protein, Gluten-Free Waffles

GLUTEN-FREE, SOY-FREE, DAIRY-FREE, VEGETARIAN

Serves 2

Per serving (*with topping*): 250 calories, 10 g fat, 25 g carbohydrate, 6 g fiber, 20 g protein

3 eggs	2 tablespoons coconut oil, melted
¼ cup coconut milk	1 teaspoon vanilla extract
1 cup almond flour	1 teaspoon pure maple syrup
¼ teaspoon sea salt	

Grease and preheat a waffle iron. In a medium bowl, whisk together eggs and coconut milk. Add almond flour and sea salt. Whisk until smooth. Add melted coconut oil and vanilla, whisking to mix well.

Scoop one-third of the batter onto the prepared waffle iron. Do not smooth the top of waffle before closing the waffle iron. Close the lid gently. Cook for approximately 5 minutes until golden brown. Serve topped with maple syrup.

Oatmeal Flapjacks

GLUTEN-FREE, SOY-FREE, DAIRY-FREE, VEGETARIAN

Serves 2

Per serving (*without topping*): 340 calories, 10 g fat, 35 g carbohydrate, 4 g fiber, 20 g protein

1 cup + 2 tablespoons gluten-free oats

¾ cup + 3 tablespoons almond or coconut milk

3 eggs

3 egg whites

1 teaspoon cinnamon

1 teaspoon coconut oil

Mix together oats, almond milk, eggs and egg whites, and cinnamon in a bowl. Heat coconut oil in a frying pan over low heat. Pour half the batter into the pan and cook until the flapjack bottom is golden, then flip and continue cooking until the reverse side is also golden. Transfer to a 250°F oven to keep warm while you cook the remaining flapjack.

Serve topped with blueberries and honey or maple syrup.

Salmon and Broccoli Frittata

GLUTEN-FREE, SOY-FREE, DAIRY-FREE

Serves 4

Per serving: 440 calories, 21 g fat, 18 g carbohydrate, 6 g fiber, 34 g protein

2 skinless wild salmon fillets
(3 ounces each)

3 new potatoes, scrubbed

1 small head broccoli, cut into
florets

1 tablespoon extra-virgin olive oil

Small handful of mint, finely
chopped

Sea salt and freshly ground black
pepper

8 eggs, beaten

Preheat the oven to 350°F. Bake salmon fillets for 25 minutes or until flakes easily when tested with a fork.

Meanwhile, boil potatoes in a large pot for 10 to 12 minutes, adding broccoli pieces for the final 4 minutes of cooking. (Potatoes and broccoli should both be tender when cooked.) Drain well.

Heat oil in a frying pan over high heat. Cut potatoes into chunky slices, then cook in the pan until golden at the edges, about 4 to 5 minutes. Reduce the heat to low, then flake the baked salmon into large chunks and place in the pan along with broccoli, among potatoes. Stir mint, sea salt, and pepper into beaten eggs, then pour into the pan. Let cook for 6 minutes or until the sides are set. Then increase the heat to high to set completely and brown, about 2 minutes. Cut into wedges and serve garnished with lettuce leaves on the side.

LUNCH

Chicken and Rice Soup

GLUTEN-FREE, SOY-FREE, DAIRY-FREE

Serves 4

Per serving: 285 calories, 6 g fat, 20 g carbohydrate, 4 g fiber, 25 g protein

4 cups low-sodium, gluten-free chicken broth

⅓ cup long-grain basmati rice

2 cups water

2 skinless, boneless chicken breast halves

2 garlic cloves, sliced

1 carrot, peeled and diced

1 celery stalk, diced

1 zucchini, diced

½ teaspoon dried thyme or 1 teaspoon minced fresh thyme

½ teaspoon dried parsley or 1 teaspoon minced fresh parsley

Sea salt and freshly ground black pepper

Juice of ½ lemon

Combine broth, rice, and water in a large saucepan. Set over medium heat and bring to a boil. Add chicken breasts and reduce the heat to low. Simmer, uncovered, until chicken is cooked through, 10 to 12 minutes. Using tongs, transfer chicken to a plate. Set aside to cool.

Stir garlic, carrot, celery, zucchini, thyme, and parsley into the broth mixture. Increase the heat to medium and cook until vegetables are softened and rice is tender but not mushy, about 10 minutes. Season with sea salt, pepper, and lemon juice.

Shred chicken or cut into small pieces, and add it to the simmering soup. Cook until heated through, about 5 minutes.

Vegetarian soup option: Omit chicken and substitute vegetable broth for chicken broth. Throw in more vegetables, such as tomatoes, mushrooms, peas, corn, baby spinach, or asparagus. Add organic tempeh or tofu to increase the vegetarian protein content.

Open-Faced Barbecue Turkey Sandwich

GLUTEN-FREE, SOY-FREE, DAIRY-FREE

Serves 4

Per serving: 403 calories, 8 g fat, 45 g carbohydrate, 3 g fiber, 40 g protein

1 small red onion, thinly sliced

1 cup finely shredded red cabbage

¼ cup balsamic vinegar

1 pound thickly sliced cooked turkey meat, cut into thin strips

⅔ cup barbecue sauce

¼ cup low-sodium, gluten-free chicken broth

4 slices gluten-free bread, toasted

Combine onion, cabbage, and vinegar in a medium bowl and set aside.

Combine turkey, barbecue sauce, and broth in a medium frying pan. Bring to a simmer over medium heat. Reduce heat to low; simmer, stirring often, until heated through, about 5 minutes.

Place 1 bread slice on each of 4 individual plates and spoon turkey mixture on top. Using tongs, pile pickled cabbage mixture atop turkey.

Lentil and Ham Salad

GLUTEN-FREE, SOY-FREE, DAIRY-FREE

Serves 2

Per serving: 400 calories, 15 g fat, 24 g carbohydrate, 9 g fiber, 30 g protein

SALAD

8 ounces ham, shredded

1 14-ounce can lentils, drained and rinsed

4 celery stalks, finely diced

2 carrots, finely diced

Handful of parsley, finely chopped

DRESSING

2 tablespoons olive oil

2 tablespoons balsamic vinegar

1 tablespoon water

½ teaspoon honey

1 teaspoon Dijon mustard

Pinch of sea salt and freshly ground black pepper

Combine salad ingredients in a large mixing bowl.

To make the dressing, whisk all dressing ingredients. Pour dressing over salad and toss well.

TIP: For a vegan variation of this salad that retains the sweet, smokey flavor added by the ham, replace the ham with 100% organic smoked tofu, chopped.

DINNER

Lamb and Squash Pasta

GLUTEN-FREE, SOY-FREE, DAIRY-FREE

Serves 4

Per serving: 500 calories, 15 g fat, 58 g carbohydrate, 9.5 g fiber, 27 g protein

5 cups peeled and cubed butternut squash

2 tablespoons avocado oil

Sea salt and freshly ground black pepper

½ pound ground lamb

2½ cups chopped onion

3 large garlic cloves, minced

2 teaspoons ground cumin

¼ teaspoon ground cinnamon

⅛ teaspoon cayenne pepper

1 cup canned crushed tomatoes with added puree

2 cups low-sodium, gluten-free chicken broth

1 cup brown rice penne pasta

½ cup chopped fresh cilantro, divided

Preheat the oven to 450°F. Toss squash with 1 tablespoon oil in a large bowl. Sprinkle with sea salt and pepper. Roast on a baking sheet for 30 to 35 minutes, using a spatula to turn occasionally, until tender and brown at the edges. Remove from the oven and set aside.

Heat remaining 1 tablespoon oil in a large frying pan over medium-high heat. Add lamb and onion, and sauté for 7 to 8 minutes or until lamb browns and onion softens. Add garlic, cumin, cinnamon, and cayenne, and cook, stirring constantly, for 1 minute. Stir in tomatoes, then broth, and bring to boil. Reduce heat and simmer until mixture thickens, about 5 minutes. Stir in squash. Season with sea salt and pepper.

Cook pasta in a large pot of boiling salted water, stirring occasionally, until al dente. Drain, reserving 1 cup cooking liquid. Return pasta to pot. Add lamb mixture and half of the cilantro, and toss. Add reserved cooking liquid in thirds to moisten as needed. Season with sea salt and pepper. Transfer pasta to individual bowls. Sprinkle with the remaining cilantro.

Spicy Vegetarian Chili

GLUTEN-FREE, SOY-FREE, DAIRY-FREE, VEGAN

6 servings

Per serving: 450 calories, 7 g fat, 60 g carbohydrate, 25 g fiber, 25 g protein

2 tablespoons coconut oil

1 onion, chopped

2 carrots, peeled and thinly sliced

1 red bell pepper, seeded and chopped

1 small jalapeño pepper, seeded and minced

1 28-ounce can crushed tomatoes

3 cups water

2 15-ounce cans black beans, drained and rinsed

2 15-ounce cans kidney beans, drained and rinsed

2 tablespoons white wine vinegar

5 garlic cloves, minced

2 tablespoons chili powder

1½ teaspoons ground cumin

1½ teaspoons ground coriander

½ teaspoon ground cinnamon

In a large pot, heat oil over medium-high heat. Add onion, carrots, bell pepper, and jalapeño, and sauté for 8 minutes or until onion and carrots are almost tender. Add the remaining ingredients and bring to a boil. Reduce heat to medium-high and cook, uncovered, for 20 minutes.

Stuffed Sweet Potatoes

GLUTEN-FREE, SOY-FREE, DAIRY-FREE

Serves 4

Per serving: 448 calories, 12 g fat, 57 g carbohydrate, 9 g fiber, 22 g protein

4 medium sweet potatoes

2 teaspoons extra-virgin olive oil

1/2 cup finely chopped onion

2 teaspoons finely chopped garlic

1 teaspoon ground cumin

1/2 teaspoon ground cinnamon

12 ounces lean ground beef

1/4 cup dry white wine

3/4 cup canned crushed tomatoes

1 tablespoon dried cranberries, chopped

1/4 cup sliced green olives

1 tablespoon capers

1/4 teaspoon sea salt

2 tablespoons chopped fresh cilantro

Preheat the oven to 425°F.

Pierce potatoes all over with a fork and place on a foil-lined baking sheet; bake for 50 minutes or until tender. Heat oil in a large frying pan over medium heat. Cook onion for 4 minutes or until soft. Add garlic, cumin, and cinnamon, and cook for 1 minute. Add beef and cook for 5 minutes or until meat is cooked through. Add wine and cook for 2 minutes, stirring constantly. Stir in tomatoes, cranberries, olives, capers, and sea salt; reduce heat and simmer for 5 minutes.

Slice open potatoes and mash insides with a fork. Divide beef mixture among potatoes, garnish with cilantro, and serve.

SNACKS

Apple Pie Smoothie

GLUTEN-FREE, SOY-FREE, DAIRY-FREE

Serves 1

Per serving: 340 calories, 4 g fat, 55 g carbohydrate, 6 g fiber, 30 g protein

1 cup applesauce, unsweetened

1 cup ice cubes

2 tablespoons ground flaxseed

1 tablespoon honey

1 teaspoon ground cinnamon

1 scoop vanilla protein powder (vegan or whey)

Place all ingredients except protein powder in a blender and blend on medium-high speed for 20 seconds or until smooth. Add protein powder and blend for another 10 seconds.

Banana Berry Blast Smoothie

GLUTEN-FREE, SOY-FREE, DAIRY-FREE, VEGAN

Serves 1

Per serving: 355 calories, 3 g fat, 55 g carbohydrate, 6 g fiber, 30 g protein

1 medium banana

1 cup strawberries (frozen or fresh)

1 cup coconut or almond milk

1 cup ice cubes

1 scoop strawberry protein powder (vegan or whey)

Place all ingredients except protein powder in a blender and blend on medium-high speed for 20 seconds or until smooth. Add protein powder and blend for another 10 seconds.

TIP: Smoothies are very versatile. If you prefer something a little different, replace strawberry protein powder with chocolate protein powder and add a spoonful of your favourite nut butter for a nutty, chocolate variation.

Cranberry Bars

GLUTEN-FREE, SOY-FREE, DAIRY-FREE, VEGETARIAN

Serves 8

Per serving: 240 calories, 7 g fat, 27 g carbohydrate, 5 g fiber, 20 g protein

2 cups gluten-free rolled oats

½ cup crushed walnuts

½ cup dried cranberries

4 tablespoons chia seeds

4 scoops vanilla protein powder (vegan or whey)

½ cup pure maple syrup

2 tablespoons honey

¼ teaspoon sea salt

¼ teaspoon vanilla extract

Olive oil

Preheat the oven to 350°F.

In a large bowl, combine oats, walnuts, cranberries, chia seeds, and vanilla protein. Add syrup, honey, sea salt, and vanilla. Stir to combine thoroughly.

Coat a large baking pan with olive oil and spread mixture evenly in the bottom of the dish. Bake for 10 minutes. Remove from the oven and cut into individual bars while still warm.

Exercises

I designed the protocols in this book specifically for fat-loss and muscle-building phases, and there are certain things in them that I urge you to stick to precisely: follow my recommendations for numbers of reps and sets in each workout and keep your rests between sets to a minimum. But the protocols are also flexible. You could do many possible variations of the exercises shown here. Feel free to adapt your workout based on the equipment available to you at home or in your gym. So long as you do the exercises at the maximum weight you can handle while maintaining proper form, and follow the other diet and exercise advice in this book, you will see amazing improvements.

In the coming pages, I've indicated muscles or muscle groups that the exercises target. As you perform the exercises, focus your attention on the muscles being worked. You may be surprised at how positively your body adapts to this kind of concentration.

For each exercise that follows, the first photo represents the starting position, and the second photo shows either the middle position (in which case the starting and finishing positions are the same) or the finishing position. Depending on your level of experience, and as you become comfortable with the protocols in the book, you may wish to incorporate other resistance-training exercises. You've got to keep challenging yourself in your workouts and vary your workout routines to keep seeing results. Just remember, consult with your primary health practitioner and a certified trainer before starting a workout routine, and if you are uncertain about how to do an exercise, ask a professional.

Now let's get to work!

LYING HIP EXTENSION

MUSCLE GROUPS: *Gluteus maximus (glutes), hamstrings, lower back*

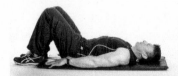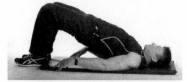

Start on the floor or a mat, lying on your back with your arms at either side, knees bent, feet hip width apart. Raise your torso by extending your hips upward while activating your glutes. Return to the starting position by lowering your torso back to the floor.

BIRD DOG

MUSCLE GROUPS: *Works everything, especially glutes, abdominals (abs), lower back, and hip muscles*

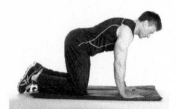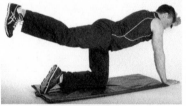

On your hands and knees with palms flat on the floor and shoulder width apart, knees hip width apart, engage your abs to stabilize and then raise your right arm and left leg at the same time until they are parallel to the floor or just higher. Return to the starting position and repeat with the left arm and right leg.

Y SQUAT

MUSCLE GROUPS: *Glutes, quadriceps (quads), upper back*

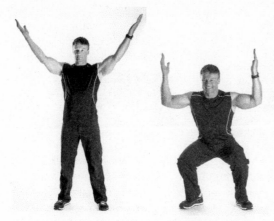

Raise your arms overhead forming a Y and then bend your knees deeply, sending your hips back, to lower into a squat. Keep your back as straight as possible. Return to the starting position by engaging the buttocks and pressing upward.

SPLIT SQUAT WITH DUMBBELLS

MUSCLE GROUPS: *Quads, glutes, hamstrings*

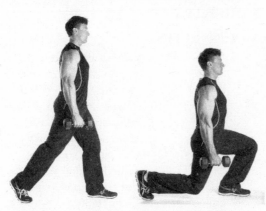

Stand with your right foot in front of your left foot. Depending on how flexible your hip flexor is, you may have your feet closer together (less flexible) or farther apart (more flexible). Bend your right leg, keeping your knee in line with your foot, until the knee of left leg is almost in contact with floor. Return to the one-legged standing position by straightening your forward leg. Repeat for the designated number of reps on the right side before switching to the left leg.

FLAT BENCH DUMBBELL CHEST PRESS

MUSCLE GROUPS: *Pectorals (pecs), triceps*

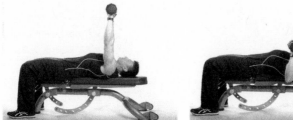

Start lying on a flat bench, with your arms fully extended, perpendicular to the floor, holding dumbbells with palms facing forward. In a gentle arc movement, lower the weights until the elbows are deeply bent and the weights hover just over the upper chest. Press the dumbbells back to the starting position following the same arc pattern.

STEP-UP WITH DUMBBELLS

MUSCLE GROUPS: *Quads, glutes, hamstrings*

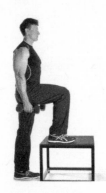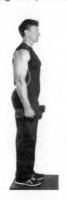

Starting with your right foot on a bench or small platform holding dumbbells at either side (if you are using weight), step up by extending the hip and knee of your right leg and placing your left foot on the bench next to the right. Step down with the left leg first, followed by the right. Repeat the entire movement, stepping up with the left leg first and down with the right leg first. This constitutes one rep.

EXERCISES

DUMBBELL ROW

MUSCLE GROUPS: *Latissimus dorsi (lats), biceps, obliques*

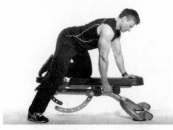 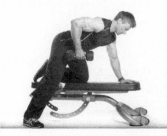

Place your left hand and knee on a flat bench with your right arm extended and holding the dumbbell in your right hand. Pull the dumbbell up to the side towards your right ribs, keeping your elbow in. Return to the start by fully extending your arm. Repeat for the designated number of reps and then perform rows on your left side.

STANDING SHOULDER PRESS WITH DUMBBELLS

MUSCLE GROUPS: *Shoulders, triceps, trapezius (traps)*

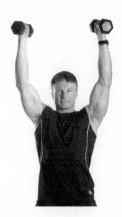 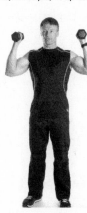

Stand, positioning the dumbbells above your head with your palms facing in. Slowly lower the dumbbells to shoulder height. Return to the starting position by pressing up the dumbbells with control.

DUMBBELL SQUAT

MUSCLE GROUPS: *Quads, glutes, hamstrings*

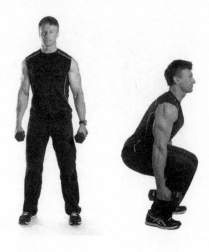

Stand with your feet shoulder width or wider apart, hands holding the dumbbells at either side. Squat down, sending your hips back while allowing your knees to move forward, keeping your back straight and your knees pointed in the same direction as your feet. Descend until your thighs are nearing parallel to the floor. Finish by extending your knees and hips until your legs are straight.

STABILITY BALL JACKKNIFE

MUSCLE GROUPS: *Works everything, especially abs*

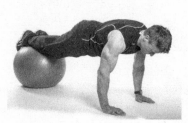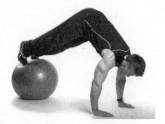

Position your feet on top of a stability ball, with your body straight and your arms in a push-up position. Flex your hips by lifting them high up until you are in an upside-down V position. Return to the starting position by lowering your hips toward the floor so that your body is in a straight line once again.

SIDE PLANK

MUSCLE GROUPS: *Obliques, glutes, shoulders*

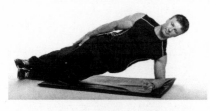

On a mat or the floor, place your right elbow under your right shoulder with your forearm perpendicular to your body. Stack your right leg and foot on top of your left and straighten both legs, lifting your legs, hips, and torso away from the floor. Hold the position for the designated amount of time (30, 60, or 90 seconds) and repeat on the left side.

BARBELL DEAD LIFT

MUSCLE GROUPS: *Quads, glutes, hamstrings*

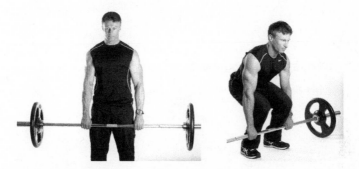

The dead lift with barbell is a more advanced version of the dead lift with dumbbells shown on page 273. A barbell dead lift puts more emphasis on the glutes as it pushes the hips farther back.

Start standing with straight legs, feet hip-width apart or wider, holding the barbell in front of you with an overhand grip, hands shoulder width apart. Lower the bar toward the floor by flexing at your hips and sending them backward in space. Bend your knees deeply during your descent and keep your waist straight so that your back is nearing parallel to floor at the lowest position. Return to upright by straightening your hips and knees. Throughout the lift, keep your arms and back straight.

PULL-UP

MUSCLE GROUPS: *Lats, biceps, shoulders*

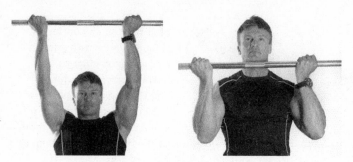

Start with your arms fully extended and with a shoulder-width grip on the horizontal bar, palms toward you with your feet off the ground. Flexing at your elbows, pull yourself up until your chin is above the bar. Return to the starting position by lowering until your arms are fully extended.

TRICEPS DIP

MUSCLE GROUPS: *Chest, triceps, shoulders*

Place your hands with palms facing inward on dip bars. Start with arms straight and shoulders above hands. Flexing at your elbows, lower your body until a stretch is felt in your shoulders. Finish by fully extending your arms.

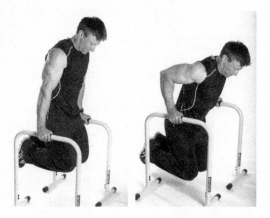

CLOSE GRIP PUSH-UP

MUSCLE GROUPS: *Triceps, chest, shoulders*

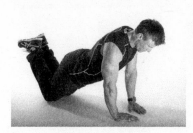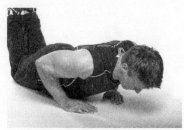

Start in a classic push-up position but with your hands slightly narrower than shoulder width apart, knees on the floor. With your body straight, lower toward the floor by bending your arms until they are at right angles, keeping your elbows in, near your side ribs. Finish by pushing up until your arms are once again extended. To increase the difficulty, work with your legs straight.

BARBELL SQUAT

MUSCLE GROUPS: *Quads, glutes, hamstrings*

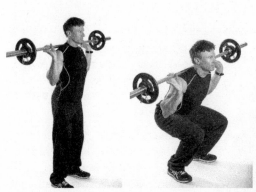

The barbell squat is a more advanced version of the dumbbell squat (page 262) because loading the body higher up puts more strain on your core muscles (hips, lower abs, glutes), making them work harder.

Start standing with the barbell high on the back of your shoulders, holding the bar with a wide grip. Squat down by bending your hips back while allowing your knees to move forward in the same direction as your feet. Keep your back straight. Descend until your thighs are close to, at, or just past parallel to the floor. Finish by straightening your legs.

EXERCISES

STANDING SHOULDER PRESS WITH BARBELL

MUSCLE GROUPS: *Shoulders, traps, triceps*

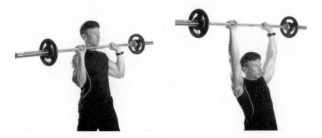

A staggered stance is preferred to help with balance in this more challenging version of the standing shoulder press with dumbbells (page 261).

Hold the barbell with hands slightly wider than shoulder width apart in an overhand grip, the barbell positioned under your chin. Press the bar upward until your arms are fully extended overhead. Lower with control to the starting position.

LUNGE WITH DUMBBELLS

MUSCLE GROUPS: *Quads, glutes, hamstrings*

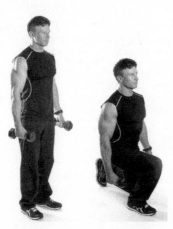

These lunges look very similar to a split squat (page 259), but the approach is slightly different as you will be stepping back to the starting position and alternating legs within a single rep.

Start standing with your feet hip width apart, holding dumbbells at either side. Step forward with your right leg. Keeping your torso straight and your right knee and foot in line, lower into the lunge by flexing the knee and hip of your right leg until your left knee is almost in contact with the floor. Step back to the starting position and repeat on the left leg. Performing this exercise on both sides constitutes one rep.

INVERTED ROW

MUSCLE GROUPS: *Lats, biceps*

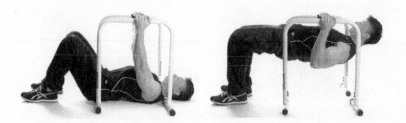

Lie on your back under exercise bars. Start with your hips lifted away from the floor, hands grasping the bars with your palms facing inward. Keep your body straight, with your knees bent or, for more challenge, legs fully extended. Pull up until your chest hovers just under the bars. Extend your arms with control to return to the starting position.

LAT PULL-DOWN

MUSCLE GROUPS: *Lats*

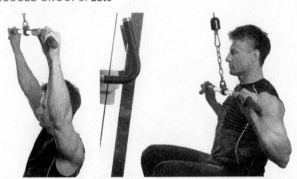

With this exercise you will need the pull-down machine. Sitting with your thighs under support, grasp the cable bar with a wide grip. Pull down the cable bar to your upper chest and return to the start by fully extending your arms.

INCLINE BENCH PRONE DUMBBELL ROWS

MUSCLE GROUPS: *Back, biceps*

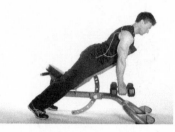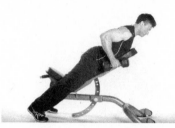

Start leaning into an incline bench with a dumbbell in each hand, your arms hanging straight down. Retract the shoulder blades and flex the elbows to pull the dumbbells to your sides. Return to the starting position by straightening your arms.

SEATED DUMBBELL ARNOLD PRESS

MUSCLE GROUPS: *Shoulders, traps, triceps*

Start with dumbbells positioned in front of your shoulders, palms facing you and your elbows under your wrists. Press the weights upward in an arc, rotating your wrists so that you finish the movement with one end of each weight touching the other overhead, palms facing away 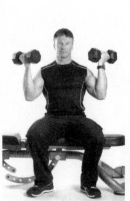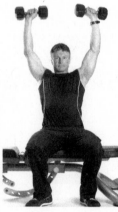 from you. Lower the weights to the front of your shoulders, reversing the movement, to return to the starting position.

SEATED LATERAL RAISE

MUSCLE GROUPS: *Shoulders, traps*

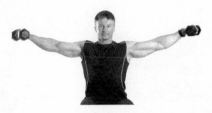
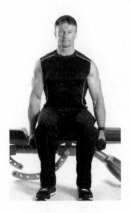

Sitting on the edge of a bench with your torso erect, hold the dumbbells at either side with your palms facing inward. Raise your arms straight out to either side until they reach shoulder height.

REVERSE CRUNCH

MUSCLE GROUPS: *Abs*

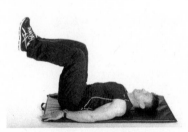
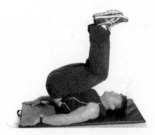

Lying on the floor or a mat, face up with your arms at your sides, palms on the floor, position your legs so that your thighs are perpendicular to the floor, calves are parallel to the floor, and legs and feet are together. Roll up your spine as you move your legs toward your torso and raise your hips off the floor. At the end of this movement your knees will be touching your chest, and your hips will be high in the air. Move with control back to the starting position.

EXERCISES

INCLINE CRUNCH ON STABILITY BALL

MUSCLE GROUPS: *Abs*

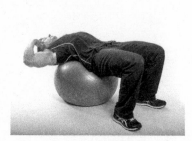 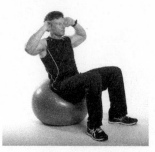

Start lying on a stability ball with your hands behind your head, your upper torso hanging off the top of the ball. Your lower back should be pressed against the ball's spherical surface, legs bent at the knee, and feet pressed firmly into the floor. With your hips stationary, flex the waist by contracting the abdominals and curl the shoulders and trunk upward so you come to an inclined seated position on the ball. Lower with control to the starting position.

ABDOMINAL KNEE TUCK ON STABILITY BALL

MUSCLE GROUPS: *Works everything, especially abs, hip flexors, upper body*

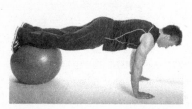 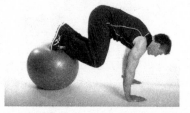

Unlike in the stability ball jackknife (page 262), in this exercise your hips stay low (but don't let them sag toward the floor).

Start in a push-up plank position with your shins resting on a stability ball and your arms straight. Pull the ball toward your chest while you draw your abs in and up, and return to the starting position by straightening your legs. Keep your upper body still throughout.

LYING TRICEPS EXTENSION WITH DUMBBELLS

MUSCLE GROUPS: *Triceps*

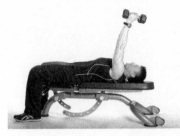 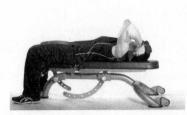

Start lying on a flat bench while holding two dumbbells with your arms fully extended perpendicular to your torso, palms facing in. Keep your upper arms stationary and the elbows in, and slowly lower the weight until the dumbbells are near your ears. Finish by bringing the weights back up above your chest, without letting the elbows splay out.

SEATED OVERHEAD DUMBBELL EXTENSION

MUSCLE GROUPS: *Triceps*

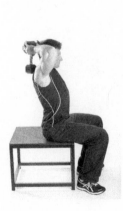 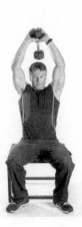

Start holding a dumbbell behind your head, with your upper arms hugging in. Raise the dumbbell up so your arms are straight. Your upper arms should remain stationary and only the forearms should move. Lower with control back to the starting position.

STANDING BICEP CURL
(REVERSE GRIP USING AN EZ CURL BAR)

MUSCLE GROUPS: *Biceps*

Start standing up straight while holding an EZ curl bar in an overhand grip at the wide outer handle, elbows close to your torso. While keeping your upper arms stationary, curl the weight up until your arms are just past 90 degrees. Slowly lower the bar back to the starting position.

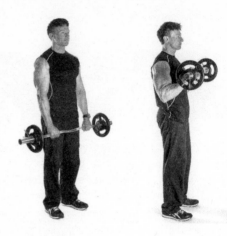

INCLINE DUMBBELL HAMMER CURL

MUSCLE GROUPS: *Biceps*

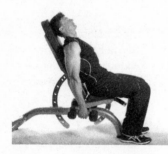
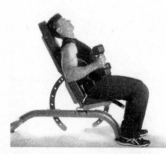

Sit on an incline bench with a dumbbell in each hand, allowing them to hang straight down at either side. Flex at the elbow until your arms form right angles, and attempt to keep the upper arm stationary. Return to the start position.

PREACHER CURL WITH STABILITY BALL

MUSCLE GROUPS: *Biceps*

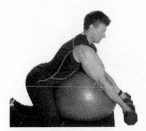
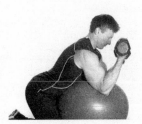

Start kneeling with your upper arms resting on a stability ball, dumbbells in an underhand grip. Keeping your lower back in its natural curve toward the ball, and without moving your upper arms off the ball, curl the dumbbells as close to your shoulders as possible. Lower to the starting position with control.

DUMBBELL DEAD LIFTS

MUSCLE GROUPS: *Hamstrings, hips, glutes*

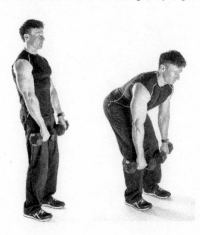

This is a more moderate version of the dead lift with barbell (page 263).

Stand with your feet shoulder width apart, holding the dumbbells in front of your thighs. Slowly lean forward, sending your hips back. Keep a moderate bend in your knees, lowering the dumbbells halfway toward the floor. Finish by returning to standing upright.

LEG CURL WITH STABILITY BALL

MUSCLE GROUPS: *Hamstrings, glutes, calves*

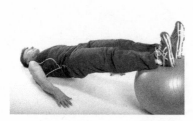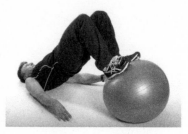

Start lying supine on the floor with arms at your sides, palms facing down, lower legs or ankles on an exercise ball, with your lower back, butt, and legs lifted off the floor. Keeping hips and lower back straight, bend your knees, pulling heels toward your rear end. Allow feet to roll up onto the ball. Lower to the starting position by straightening your legs.

STANDING CALF RAISE

MUSCLE GROUPS: *Calves*

Start standing on a bench (or another platform, for example stairs) with the balls of your feet placed securely on top, toes facing forward, heels off the bench. With legs straight, raise your heels by extending your ankles as high as possible. To return to the starting position, lower your heels as you bend the ankles until calves are stretched. Use a hand on a wall or rail to help with balance if necessary.

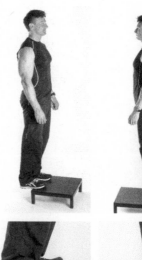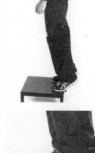

DUMBBELL PULLOVER

MUSCLE GROUPS: *Lats, chest*

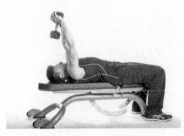 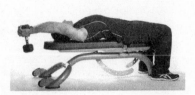

Start lying on a flat bench with arms perpendicular to the floor and fully straight, both hands holding the weight above your head. Lower the dumbbell over and beyond your head until your upper arms are in line with your torso. Finish by pulling the dumbbell back up to the starting position with your arms perpendicular to your body.

INCLINE DUMBBELL FLY

MUSCLE GROUPS: *Upper chest*

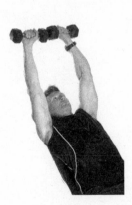 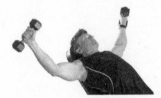

Start sitting on an incline bench, with dumbbells touching above your head, arms straight. Open the dumbbells out to the sides. Finish by lifting the weights with straight arms back overhead.

BARBELL REVERSE GRIP BENT-OVER ROWS

MUSCLE GROUPS: *Lats, biceps*

Start holding barbell in an underhand grip, your hips flexed so your torso bends over the bar. Have your knees slightly bent. Pull the bar up to your waist. Return to the starting position by extending your arms.

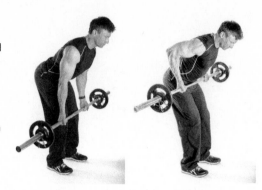

SELECTED SOURCES

Arima, H., Y. Kiyohara, I. Kato, Y. Tanizaki, M. Kubo, H. Iwamoto, K. Tanaka, I. Abe, and M. Fujishima. 2002. "Alcohol reduces insulin-hypertension relationship in a general population: the Hisayama study." *Journal of Clinical Epidemiology* 55 (9): 863–69. http://www.ncbi.nlm.nih.gov/pubmed/12393073.

Buitrago, S., N. Wirtz, Z. Yue, H. Kleinöder, and J. Mester. 2012. "Effects of load and training modes on physiological and metabolic responses in resistance exercise." *European Journal of Applied Physiology* 112 (7): 2739–48.

Christensen, R., J. K. Lorenzen, C. R. Svith, E. M. Bartels, E. L. Melanson, W. H. Saris, A. Tremblay, and A. Astrup. 2009. "Effect of calcium from dairy and dietary supplements on faecal fat excretion: a meta-analysis of randomized controlled trials." *Obesity Reviews* 10 (4): 475–86. doi: 10.1111/j.1467-789X.2009.00599.

Cinar, V., A. K. Baltaci, R. Moqulkoc, and M. Kilic. 2009. "Testosterone levels in athletes at rest and exhaustion: effects of calcium supplementation." *Biological Trace Element Research* 129 (103): 65–69. doi: 10.1007/s12011-008-8294-5.

Crum, A. J., W. R. Corbin, K. D. Brownell, and P. Salovey. 2011. "Mind over milkshakes: mindsets, not just nutrients, determine ghrelin response." *Health Psychology* 30 (4): 424–29. doi: 10.1037/a0023467.

De Martino, B., D. Kumaran, B. Seymour, and R. J. Dolan. 2006.

"Frames, biases, and rational decision-making in the human brain." *Science* 313 (5787): 684–87. doi: 10.1126/science.1128356.

Dreon, D. M., H. A. Fernstrom, H. Campos, P. Blanche, P. T. Williams, and R. M. Krauss. 1998. "Change in dietary saturated fat intake is correlated with change in mass of large low-density-lipoprotein particles in men." *American Journal of Clinical Nutrition* 67 (5): 828–36. http://ajcn.nutrition.org/content/67/5/828.short.

Evans, K., M. L. Clark, and K. N. Frayn. 1999. "Effects of an oral and intravenous fat load on adipose tissue and forearm lipid metabolism." *American Journal of Physiology* 276 (2, pt. 1): 241–48. http://www.ncbi.nlm.nih.gov/pubmed/9950782.

Fischer-Posovszky, P., V. Kukulus, M. A. Zulet, K. M. Debatin, and M. Wabitsch. 2007. "Conjugated linoleic acids promote human fat cell apoptosis." *Hormonal Metabolic Research* 39 (3): 186–91. http://www.ncbi.nlm.nih.gov/pubmed/17373632.

Fry, A. C., R. Kudrna, P. M. Gallagher, N. Moodie, and M. Prewitt. 2011. "Acute endocrine responses to maximal velocity barbell squats with three different loads." *Journal of Strength and Conditioning Research* 25 (8): S91–S92. doi: 10.1097/01.JSC.0000395724.29988.94.

Gaziano, J. M., T. A. Gaziano, R. J. Glynn, H. D. Sesso, U. A. Ajani, M. J. Stampfer, J. E. Manson, C. H. Hennekens, and J. E. Buring. 2000. "Light-to-moderate alcohol consumption and mortality in the Physicians' Health Study enrollment cohort." *Journal of the American College of Cardiology* 35 (1): 96–105. http://www.ncbi.nlm.nih.gov/pubmed/10636266.

Gravholt, C. H., N. Møller, M. D. Jensen, J. S. Christiansen, and O. Schmitz. 2001. "Physiological levels of glucagon do not influence lipolysis in abdominal adipose tissue as assessed by microdialysis." *Journal of Clinical Endocrinology and Metabolism* 86 (5): 2085–89. http://www.ncbi.nlm.nih.gov/pubmed/11344211.

Henderson, G. C., J. A. Fattor, M. A. Horning, N. Faghihnia, M. L. Johnson, T. L. Mau, M. Luke-Zeitoun, and G. A. Brooks. 2007. "Lipolysis and fatty acid metabolism in men and women during postexercise recovery period." *Journal of Physiology* 584 (3): 963–81. doi: 10.1113/jphysiol.2007.137331.

Holt, S. H., J. C. Miller, and P. Petocz. 1997. "An insulin index of foods: the insulin demand generated by 1000-kJ portions of common foods." *American Journal of Clinical Nutrition* 66 (5): 1264–76. http://www.ncbi.nlm.nih.gov/pubmed/9356547.

Horton, T. J., M. J. Pagliassotti, K. Hobbs, and J. O. Hill. 1998. "Fuel metabolism in men and women during and after long-duration exercise." *Journal of Applied Physiology* 85 (5): 1823–32. http://jap.physiology.org/content/85/5/1823.

Joslin Diabetes Center. "'Good fat' activated by cold, not ephedrine." *ScienceDaily.* www.sciencedaily.com/releases/2012/06/120604155556.htm. Accessed June 18, 2014.

Keim, N. L., M. D. Van Loan, W. F. Horn, T. F. Barbieri, and P. L. Mayclin. 1997. "Weight loss is greater with consumption of large morning meals and fat-free mass is preserved with large evening meals in women on a controlled weight reduction regimen." *Journal of Nutrition* 127 (1): 75–82. http://www.ncbi.nlm.nih.gov/pubmed/9040548.

Kershaw, E. E., and J. S. Flier. 2004. "Adipose tissue as an endocrine organ." *Journal of Clinical Endocrinology & Metabolism* 89 (6): 2548–56. doi: 10.1210/jc.2004-0395.

Kersten, S. 2001. "Mechanisms of nutritional and hormonal regulation of lipogenesis." *EMBO Reports* 2 (4): 282–86. doi: 0.1093/embo-reports/kve071.

Kraemer, B. F., and W.-J. Shen. 2002. "Hormone-sensitive lipase: control of intracellular tri-(di-)acylglycerol and cholesteryl ester hydrolysis." *Journal of Lipid Research* 43 (10): 1585–94. doi: 10.1194/jlr.R200009-JLR200.

Leidy, H. J., C. L. Armstrong, M. Tang, R. D. Mattes, and W. W. Campbell. 2010. "The influence of higher protein intake and greater eating frequency on appetite control in overweight and obese men." *Obesity* (Silver Spring) 18 (9): 1725–32. doi: 10.1038/oby.2010.45.

Lund, S., G. D. Holman, O. Schmitz, and O. Pedersen. 1995. "Contraction stimulates translocation of glucose transporter GLUT4 in skeletal muscle through a mechanism distinct from that of insulin." *Proceedings of the National Academy of Sciences* 92 (13): 5817–21. doi: 10.1073/pnas.92.13.5817.

Mader, I., M. Wabitsch, K.-M. Debatin, P. Fischer-Posovszky, and S. Fulda. 2010. "Identification of a novel proapoptotic function of resveratrol in fat cells: SIRT1-independent sensitization to TRAIL-induced apoptosis." *FASEB Journal* 24 (1): 1–13. http://www.fasebj.org/content/early/2010/01/22/fj.09-142943.full.pdf.

McCaulley, G., J. McBride, P. Cormie, M. Hudson, J. Nuzzo, J. Quidry, and N. Triplett. 2009. "Acute hormonal and neuromuscular responses to hypertrophy, strength and power type resistance exercise." *European Journal of Applied Physiology* 105 (5): 695–704.

Meckel, Y., A. Eliakim, F. Seraev, F. Zaldivar, D. Cooper, M. Sabiv, and D. Nemet. 2009. "The effect of a brief sprint interval exercise on growth factors and inflammatory mediators." *Journal of Strength and Conditioning Research* 23 (1): 225–30.

Meckel, Y., D. Nemet, S. Bar-Sela, S. Radom-Aizik, D. M. Cooper, M. Sagiv, and A. Eliakim. 2011. "Hormonal and inflammatory responses to different types of sprint interval training." *Journal of Strength and Conditioning Research* 25 (8): 2161–69. doi: 10.1519/JSC.0b013e3181dc4571.

Meo, S. A., A. M. Al-Drees, S. Husain, M. M. Khan, and M. B. Imran. 2010. "Effects of mobile phone radiation on serum testosterone in Wistar albino rats." *Saudi Medical Journal* 31 (8): 869–73. http://www.ncbi.nlm.nih.gov/pubmed/20714683.

Miller, M. D., K. M. Crofton, D. C. Rice, and R. Thomas Zoeller. 2009. "Thyroid-disrupting chemicals: interpreting upstream biomarkers of adverse outcomes." *Environmental Health Perspectives* 117 (7): 1033–41. doi: 10.1289/ehp.0800247.

Millet, L., P. Barbe, M. Lafontan, M. Berlan, and J. Galitzky. 1998. "Catecholamine effects on lipolysis and blood flow in human abdominal and femoral adipose tissue." *Journal of Applied Physiology* 85 (1): 181–88. http://jap.physiology.org/content/jap/85/1/181.

Nguyen, T. T., A. H. Mijares, C. M. Johnson, and M. D. Jensen. 1996. "Postprandial leg and splanchnic fatty acid metabolism in nonobese men and women." *American Journal of Physiology—Endocrinology*

and Metabolism 271 (6): 965–72. http://ajpendo.physiology.org
/content/271/6/E965.

Orwell, S., and K. Frank. "New uses for creatine." *T Nation*. http://
www.t-nation.com/free_online_article/most_recent/new_uses
_for_creatine. Accessed June 18, 2014.

Ouellet, V., S. M. Labbé, D. P. Blondin, S. Phoenix, B. Guérin, F.
Haman, E. E. Turcotte, D. Richard, and A. C. Carpentier. 2012.
"Brown adipose tissue oxidative metabolism contributes to energy
expenditure during acute cold exposure in humans." *Journal of
Clinical Investigation* 122 (2): 545–52. doi: 10.1172/JCI60433.

Packard, C., M. Caslake, and J. Shepherd. 2000. "The role of small, dense
low density lipoprotein (LDL): a new look." *International Journal of
Cardiology* 74 (1): 15–22. doi: 10.1016/S0167-5273(99)00107-2.

Pedersen, S. B., K. Kristensen, P. A. Hermann, J. A. Katzenellenbogen,
and B. Richelsen. 2004. "Estrogen controls lipolysis by up-regulating
alpha2A-adrenergic receptors directly in human adipose tissue
through the estrogen receptor alpha: implications for the female
fat distribution." *Journal of Clinical Endocrinology and Metabolism* 89
(4): 1869–78. http://www.ncbi.nlm.nih.gov/pubmed/15070958.

Rashidkhani, B., A. Akesson, P. Lindblad, and A. Wolk. 2005. "Alcohol
consumption and risk of renal cell carcinoma: a prospective study
of Swedish women." *International Journal of Cancer* 117 (5): 848–53.
http://www.ncbi.nlm.nih.gov/pubmed/15957170.

Romanski, S. A., R. M. Nelson, and M. D. Jensen. 2000. "Meal fatty
acid uptake in adipose tissue: gender effects in nonobese humans."
American Journal of Physiology—Endocrinology and Metabolism 279 (2):
455–62. http://ajpendo.physiology.org/content/279/2/E455.

Rosenow, A., T. N. Arrey, F. G. Bouwman, J.-P. Noben, M. Wabitsch,
E. C. M. Mariman, M. Karas, and J. Renes. 2010. "Identification
of novel human adipocyte secreted proteins by using SGBS cells."
Journal of Proteome Research 9 (10): 5389–401. doi: 10.1021/pr100621g.

Samra, J. S., M. L. Clark, S. M. Humphreys, I. A. Macdonald, and
K. N. Frayn. 1996. "Regulation of lipid metabolism in adipose
tissue during early starvation." *American Journal of Physiology* 271
(3, pt. 1): 541–46. http://www.ncbi.nlm.nih.gov/pubmed/8843749.

Shapiro A., N. Tümer, Y. Gao, K. Y. Cheng, and P. J. Scarpace. 2011. "Prevention and reversal of diet-induced leptin resistance with a sugar-free diet despite high fat content." *British Journal of Nutrition* 106 (3): 390–97. doi: 10.1017/S000711451100033X.

Siri-Tarino, P. W., Q. Sun, F. B. Hu, and R. M. Krauss. 2010. "Meta-analysis of prospective cohort studies evaluating the association of saturated fat with cardiovascular disease." *American Journal of Clinical Nutrition* 91 (3): 1–12. doi: 10.3945/ajcn.2009.27725.

Stallknecht, B., F. Dela, and J. Wulff Helge. 2007. "Are blood flow and lipolysis in subcutaneous adipose tissue influenced by contractions in adjacent muscles in humans?" *American Journal of Physiology —Endocrinology and Metabolism* 292 (2): 394–99. doi: 10.1152/ajpendo.00215.2006.

Stote, K. S., D. J. Baer, K. Spears, D. R. Paul, G. K. Harris, W. V. Rumpler, P. Strycula, S. S. Najjar, L. Ferrucci, D. K. Ingram, D. L. Longo, and M. P. Mattson. 2007. "A controlled trial of reduced meal frequency with caloric restriction in healthy, normal-weight, middle-aged adults." *American Journal of Clinical Nutrition* 85 (4): 981–88. http://www.ncbi.nlm.nih.gov/pubmed/17413096.

Valle, A., B. Català-Niell, B. Colom, F. J. García-Palmer, J. Oliver, and P. Roca. 2005. "Sex-related differences in energy balance in response to caloric restriction." *American Journal of Physiology—Endocrinology and Metabolism* 289 (1): 15–22. doi: 10.1152/ajpendo.00553.2004.

Van Marken Lichtenbelt, W. D., J. W. Vanhommerig, N. M. Smulders, J. M. A. F. L. Drossaerts, G. J. Kenerink, N. D. Bouvy, P. Shrauwen, and G. J. Jaap Teule. 2009. "Cold-activated brown adipose tissue in healthy men." *New England Journal of Medicine* 360 (15): 1500–08. http://www.nejm.org/doi/pdf/10.1056/NEJMoa0808718.

Vella, C. A., and L. Kravitz. 2002. "Gender differences in fat metabolism." *IDEA Health & Fitness Source* 2003 (10). http://www.ideafit.com/fitness-library/gender-differences-fat-metabolism.

ACKNOWLEDGEMENTS

First and foremost, I thank God for all that I am, all that I have, and all that I will ever be. I hand over all glory to you.

Certainly, my greatest blessing has been my wife, Janet, without whom I could never hope to achieve or even dream to achieve all that I have. I love you.

Thanks to all the great researchers, trailblazers, and forward thinkers who paved the road for this book to follow. This includes (but is certainly not limited to) John Berardi, Charles Poliquin, Tom Venuto, Lyle McDonald, Martin Berkhan, Brad Pilon, James Krieger, Joseph Mercola, Alan Aragon, and Sam Graci. Your brilliant minds light up the health and fitness world.

Thanks to my clients, who put up with my endless rants about training and nutrition (and unwittingly serve as guinea pigs).

Thanks to my agent Hilary McMahon and the great people at Appetite (including Robert McCullough and my very talented editor, Kendra Ward) who believed in the project from the beginning.

Thanks to my Christian brothers, who have lifted me up and supported me—Luciano, Vince, Shaun, Dan, Chad, Joel, Ryan, Mike, and the rest of the fit pro group—you guys are awesome.

Thanks to you, the reader, for investing in this book—I pray that it is the answer you have been searching for.

INDEX